PROGRESS IN CLINICAL AND BIOLOGICAL RESEARCH

Series Editors

RECENT TITLES

Vol 336: **Dynamic Interactions of Myelin Proteins,** George A. Hashim, Mario Moscarello, *Editors*

Vol 337: **Apheresis,** Gail Rock, Editor

Vol 338: **Hematopoietic Growth Factors in Transfusion Medicine,** Jerry Spivak, William Drohan, Douglas Dooley, *Editors*

Vol 339: **Advances in Cancer Control: Screening and Prevention Research,** Paul F. Engstrom, Barbara Rimer, Lee E. Mortenson, *Editors*

Vol 340: **Mutation and the Environment,** Mortimer L. Mendelsohn, Richard J. Albertini, *Editors*. Published in five volumes: *Part A: Basic Mechanisms. Part B: Metabolism, Testing Methods, and Chromosomes. Part C: Somatic and Heritable Mutation, Adduction, and Epidemiology. Part D: Carcinogenesis. Part E: Environmental Genotoxicity, Risk, and Modulation.*

Vol 341: **Chronobiology: Its Role in Clinical Medicine, General Biology, and Agriculture,** Dora K. Hayes, John E. Pauly, Russel J. Reiter, *Editors*. Published in two volumes.

Vol 342: **Progress in Comparative Endocrinology,** August Epple, Colin G. Scanes, Milton H. Stetson, *Editors*

Vol 343: **Horizons in Membrane Biotechnology,** Claude Nicolau, Dennis Chapman, *Editors*

Vol 344: **Isozymes: Structure, Function, and Use in Biology and Medicine,** Zen-Ichi Ogita, Clement L. Markert, *Editors*

Vol 345: **Sleep and Respiration,** Faiq G. Issa, Paul M. Suratt, John E. Remmers, *Editors*

Vol 346: **Recent Progress in Research on Nutrition and Cancer,** Curtis J. Mettlin, Kunio Aoki, *Editors*

Vol 347: **Mutagens and Carcinogens in the Diet,** Michael W. Pariza, Hans-Ulrich Aeschbacher, James S. Felton, Shigeaki Sato, *Editors*

Vol 348: **EORTC Genitourinary Group Monograph 9: Basic Research and Treatment of Renal Cell Carcinoma Metastasis,** C.G. Bollack, D. Jacqmin, *Editors*

Vol 349: **Cytokines and Lipocortins in Inflammation and Differentiation,** Marialuisa Melli, Luca Parente, *Editors*

Vol 350: **Uro-Oncology: Current Status and Future Trends,** H.G.W. Frohmüller, Manfred Wirth, *Editors*

Vol 351: **Taurine: Functional Neurochemistry, Physiology, and Cardiology,** Herminia Pasantes-Morales, David L. Martin, William Shain, Rafael Martín del Río, *Editors*

Vol 352: **The Biology of Hematopoiesis,** Nicholas Daniak, Eugene P. Cronkite, Ronald McCaffrey, Richard K. Shadduck, *Editors*

Vol 353: **Neoadjuvant Chemotherapy in Invasive Bladder Cancer,** Ted A.W. Splinter, Howard I. Scher, *Editors*

Vol 354: **Effects of Therapy on Biology and Kinetics of the Residual Tumor,** Joseph Ragaz, Linda Simpson-Herren, Marc Lippman, Bernard Fisher, *Editors*. Published in two volumes: *Part A: Pre-Clinical Aspects. Part B: Clinical Aspects.*

Vol 355: **Radiolabelled Cellular Blood Elements,** Helmut Sinzinger, Mathew L. Thakur, *Editors*

Vol 356: **Molecular Biology and Differentiation of Megakaryocytes,** Janine Breton-Gorius, Jack Levin, Alan T. Nurden, Neil Williams, *Editors*

Vol 357: **EORTC Genitourinary Group Monograph 7: Prostate Cancer and Testicular Cancer,** Donald W.W. Newling, William G. Jones, *Editors*

Vol 358: **Treatment of Post Surgical Adhesions,** Gere S. diZerega, L. Russell Malinak, Michael P. Diamond, Cary B. Linsky, *Editors*

Vol 359: **EORTC Genitourinary Group Monograph 8: Treatment of Prostatic Cancer—Facts and Controversies,** Fritz H. Schröder, *Editor*

Vol 360: **Molecular Genetics of Chromosome 21 and Down Syndrome,** David Patterson, Charles J. Epstein, *Editors*

Vol 361: **Current and Future Trends in Anticonvulsant, Anxiety, and Stroke Therapy,** Brian S. Meldrum, Michael Williams, *Editors*

Vol 362: **The Molecular Biology of the Retina: Basic and Clinically Relevant Studies,** Debora B. Farber, Gerald J. Chader, *Editors*

Vol 363: **Information Processing in Medical Imaging,** Douglas A. Ortendahl, Jorge Llacer, *Editors*

Vol 364: **The Hepatitis Delta Virus,** John L. Gerin, Robert H. Purcell, Mario Rizzetto, *Editors*

Vol 365: **Clinical and Experimental Approaches to Dermal and Epidermal Repair: Normal and Chronic Wounds,** Adrian Barbul, Michael D. Caldwell, William H. Eaglstein, Thomas K. Hunt, David Marshall, Eli Pines, Greg Skover, *Editors*

Vol 366: **Advances in Neuroblastoma Research 3,** Audrey E. Evans, Guilio J. D'Angio, Alfred F. Knudson, Jr., Robert C. Seeger, *Editors*

Vol 367: **Bacterial Endotoxins: Cytokine Mediators and New Therapies for Sepsis,** Auguste Sturk, Sander J.H. van Deventer, Jan Wouter ten Cate, Harry R. Büller, Lambertus G. Thijs, Jack Levin, *Editors*

Vol 368: **Fragile X/Cancer Cytogenetics,** Ann M. Willey, Patricia D. Murphy, *Editors*

Vol 369: **Chemically Induced Cell Proliferation: Implications for Risk Assessment,** Byron E. Butterworth, Thomas J. Slaga, William Farland, and Michael McClain, *Editors*

Vol 370: **EORTC Genitourinary Group Monograph 10: Urological Oncology: Reconstructive Surgery, Organ Conservation, and Restoration of Function,** Philip H. Smith and Michele Pavone-Macaluso, *Editors*

Vol 371: **Operations Research: Helping Family Planning Programs Work Better,** Myrna Seidman and Marjorie C. Horn, *Editors*

Vol 372: **New Horizons in Biological Dosimetry,** Barton L. Gledhill and Francesco Mauro, *Editors*

Vol. 373: **The Morphogenesis of Down Syndrome,** Charles J. Epstein, *Editor*

Vol 374: **Relevance of Animal Studies to the Evaluation of Human Cancer Risk,** Robert D'Amato, Thomas J. Slaga, William H. Farland, Carol Henry, *Editors*

Vol 375: **New Developments in Fatty Acid Oxidation,** Paul M. Coates and Kay Tanaka, *Editors*

Vol 376: **Comparative Molecular Carcinogenesis,** Andres J.P. Klein-Szanto, Marshall Anderson, J. Carl Barrett, Thomas J. Slaga, *Editors*

Vol 377: **Advances in Bone Marrow Purging and Processing,** Diana Worthington-White, Adrian Gee, Samuel Gross, *Editors*

Vol 378: **EORTC Genitourinary Group Monograph 11: Recent Progress in Bladder and Kidney Cancer,** Fritz H. Schröder, *Editor*

Vol 379: **Down Syndrome and Alzheimer Disease.** Lynn Nadel, Charles J. Epstein, *Editors*

Vol 380: **Essential and Toxic Trace Elements in Human Health and Disease, Vol. II,** Ananda S. Prasad, *Editor*

Vol 381: **Gynecologic Surgery and Adhesion Prevention,** Michael P. Diamond, Gere S. diZerega, Cary B. Linsky, Robert L. Reid, *Editors*

Vol 382: **Hepatitis Delta Virus: Molecular Biology, Pathogenesis, and Clinical Aspects,** Stephanos J. Hadziyannis, John M. Taylor, Ferruccio Bonino, *Editors*

Vol 383: **Limb Development and Regeneration, Parts A and B,** John F. Fallon, Paul F. Goetinck, Robert O. Kelley, David L. Slocum, *Editors*

Please contact the publisher for information about previous titles in this series

GYNECOLOGIC SURGERY AND ADHESION PREVENTION

GYNECOLOGIC SURGERY AND ADHESION PREVENTION

Proceedings of the Second International Symposium on Gynecologic Surgery and Adhesion Prevention, Held in Palm Beach, Florida, January 1992

Editors

Michael P. Diamond
Department of Obstetrics and Gynecology
Vanderbilt University Medical Center
Nashville, Tennessee

Gere S. diZerega
Department of Obstetrics and Gynecology
University of Southern California School of Medicine
Los Angeles, California

Cary B. Linsky
Department of Clinical Research
Ethicon, Inc.
Somerville, New Jersey

Robert L. Reid
Department of Obstetrics and Gynaecology
Queen's University
Kingston, Ontario, Canada

WILEY-LISS

A JOHN WILEY & SONS, INC., PUBLICATION
NEW YORK • CHICHESTER • BRISBANE • TORONTO • SINGAPORE

Address all Inquiries to the Publisher
Wiley-Liss, Inc., 605 Third Avenue, New York, NY 10158-0012

Printed in the United States of America.

While the authors, editors, and publisher believe that drug selection and dosage and the specification and usage of equipment and devices, as set forth in this book, are in accord with current recommendations and practice at the time of publication, they accept no legal responsibility for any errors or omissions, and make no warranty, express or implied, with respect to material contained herein. In view of ongoing research, equipment modifications, changes in governmental regulations and the constant flow of information relating to drug therapy, drug reactions, and the use of equipment and devices, the reader is urged to review and evaluate the information provided in the package insert or instructions for each drug, piece of equipment, or device for, among other things, any changes in the instructions or indication of dosage or usage and for added warnings and precautions.

The publication of this volume was facilitated by the authors and editors who submitted the text in a form suitable for direct reproduction without subsequent editing or proofreading by the publisher.

Library of Congress Cataloging-in-Publication Data

Gynecologic surgery and adhesion prevention / editors, Michael P. Diamond ... [et al.].
p. cm. -- (Progress in clinical and biological research ; 381)
Includes bibliographical references and index.
ISBN 0-471-58832-6
1. Generative organs, Female—Surgery—Complications—Prevention. 2. Adhesions—Prevention. I. Diamond, Michael P. II. Series: Progress in clinical and biological research ; v. 381.
[DNLM: 1. Adhesions—prevention & control. 2. Postoperative Complications—prevention & control. 3. Genital Diseases, Female--surgery. W1 PR668E v. 381 1993 / WP 140 G99717 1993]
RG104.2.G95 1993
618.1'45—dc20
DNLM/DLC
for Library of Congress 93-6849
CIP

The text of this book is printed on acid-free paper.

Contents

Contributors

G. David Adamson, Department of Gynecology and Obstetrics, Stanford University School of Medicine, Stanford, CA 94305; and Fertility and Reproductive Health Institute of Northern California, San Jose, CA 95124 **[155]**

Jacques Barbot, Hôpital St. Jaques Paris, France **[65]**

Stephen Boyers, University of California, Davis School of Medicine, Sacramento, CA 95816 **[253]**

Ivo Brosens, Department of Obstetrics and Gynaecology, Center for Surgical Technologies, University Hospital Gasthuisberg, B 3000 Leuven, Belgium **[121]**

James W. Burns, Genzyme Corporation, Cambridge, MA 02139 **[191]**

Robert F. Casper, Department of Obstetrics and Gynecology, University of Toronto, Toronto, Ontario, M5G 2C4 Canada **[129]**

James F. Daniell, Centennial Medical Center, Nashville, TN 37203 **[59]**

Michael P. Diamond, Department of Obstetrics and Gynecology, Vanderbilt University, Nashville, TN 37232 **[xiii,51,205]**

Gere S. diZerega, Department of Obstetrics and Gynecology, Livingston Reproductive Biology Laboratory, University of Southern California School of Medicine, Los Angeles County-University of Southern California Medical Center, Los Angeles, CA 90033 **[ix,1]**

Randall C. Dunn, Department of Obstetrics and Gynecology, Baylor College of Medicine, Houston, TX 77030 **[213]**

Robert Franklin, Women's Hospital of Texas and Baylor College of Medicine, Houston, TX 77054 **[253]**

Eugene P. Goldberg, Biomedical Engineering Center, Department of Materials Science and Engineering, University of Florida, Gainesville, FL 32611 **[191]**

L.E. Gottlick, Ethicon, Inc., Somerville, NJ 08876 **[205]**

Ellen Mary Greenblatt, Department of Obstetrics and Gynecology, University of Toronto, Toronto, Ontario, M5G 2C4 Canada **[129]**

Ana Griffin, Department of Obstetrics and Gynecology, Baylor College of Medicine, Houston, TX 77030-3498 **[97]**

The numbers in brackets are the opening page numbers of the contributors' articles.

Arthur F. Haney, Division of Reproductive Endocrinology and Infertility, Department of Obstetrics and Gynecology, Duke University Medical Center, Durham, NC 27710 **[19,253]**

Simon Henderson, San Francisco Center for Reproductive Medicine and the Department of Obstetrics and Gynecology, California Pacific Medical Center, San Francisco, CA 94118 **[235]**

Gary Holtz, Southeastern Fertility Center, Mt. Pleasant, SC 29464 **[81]**

Bradley Hurst, The Johns Hopkins Hospital, Baltimore, MD 21205 **[253]**

L.F. Kamp, Ethicon, Inc., Somerville, NJ 08876 **[205]**

Bryan R. Kurtz, Centennial Medical Center, Nashville, TN 37203 **[59]**

Hovey Lambert, San Francisco Center for Reproductive Medicine and the Department of Obstetrics and Gynecology, California Pacific Medical Center, San Francisco, CA 94118 **[235]**

Annette I. La Morte, Department of Obstetrics and Gynecology, Yale University School of Medicine, New Haven, CT 06510 **[51]**

Kay Lie, Department of Obstetrics and Gynaecology, University of Toronto, Toronto, Ontario, Canada **[261]**

Cary B. Linsky, Department of Clinical Research, Ethicon, Inc., Somerville, NJ 08876 **[xiii,205]**

Eberhard Lotze, Women's Hospital of Texas and Baylor College of Medicine, Houston, TX 77054 **[253]**

Per Lundorff, Department of Obstetrics and Gynecology, Sahlgrenska Hospital, Gothenburg, Sweden **[139]**

L. Russell Malinak, Department of Obstetrics and Gynecology, Baylor College of Medicine, Houston, TX 77030-3498 **[97]**

Charles M. March, University of Southern California School of Medicine, Los Angeles, CA 90033 **[253]**

Robert S. Neuwirth, Department of Hysteroscopic Surgery, College of Physicians and Surgeons of Columbia University, St. Luke's-Roosevelt Hospital Center, New York, NY 10025 **[187]**

Margaret R. Punch, Department of Obstetrics and Gynecology, University of Michigan Medical Center, Ann Arbor, MI 48109 **[101]**

Robert L. Reid, Department of Obstetrics and Gynaecology, Queen's University, Kingston, Ontario, Canada **[xiii,261]**

John A. Rock, The Johns Hopkins Hospital, Baltimore, MD 21205; present address: Department of Obstetrics and Gynecology, Emory University, Atlanta, GA **[253]**

Randy S. Roth, Departments of Anesthesiology and Physical Medicine and Rehabilitation, University of Michigan Medical Center, Ann Arbor, MI 48109 **[101]**

Guillermo Rowe, Women's Hospital of Texas and Baylor College of Medicine, Houston, TX 77054 **[253]**

L. Saferstein, Noramco, Inc., New Brunswick, NJ 08903 **[205]**

William Schalaff, University of Colorado Health Science Center, Denver, CO 80210 **[253]**

Kaoru Sekiba, Department of Obstetrics and Gynecology, Okayama University Medical School, Okayama 700, Japan **[221]**

John E. Spence, Department of Obstetrics and Gynaecology, University of Ottawa, Ottawa, Ontario, Canada **[261]**

Alex Steinleitner, San Francisco Center for Reproductive Medicine and the Department of Obstetrics and Gynecology, California Pacific Medical Center, San Francisco, CA 94118 **[235]**

Kurt Swolin, Department of Obstetrics, Sahlgrenska Hospital, The University of Göteborg, S-413 45 Göteborg, Sweden **[45]**

Togas Tulandi, Division of Reproductive Endocrinology and Infertility, Department of Obstetrics and Gynecology, McGill University, Montreal, Quebec, H3A 1A1 Canada **[149, 261]**

D.M. Wiseman, Ethicon, Inc., Somerville, NJ 08876 **[205]**

Yoseph Yaacobi, Biomedical Engineering Center, Department of Materials Science and Engineering, University of Florida, Gainesville, FL 32611 **[191]**

Albert Yuzpe, Department of Obstetrics and Gynaecology, University of Western Ontario, London, Ontario, Canada **[261]**

Preface

This book represents an updated synopsis on the status of the fight against postoperative adhesions. This field rapidly expanded between the First International Symposium for the Treatment of Postsurgical Adhesions, held in Phoenix, Arizona, in September 1989, and the Second International Symposium on Gynecologic Surgery and Adhesion Prevention, held in Palm Beach, Florida, in January 1992. The area continues to expand as more physicians become aware of the extent of the problem of postoperative adhesions. The 1992 symposium reflected this awareness through its many presentations identifying the frequency of postoperative adhesion development.

More importantly, the understanding of the pathophysiological mechanisms responsible for adhesion development is greatly expanding. These mechanisms responsible for adhesion development involve a multitude of cell-regulating systems. The surgical armamentarium to combat adhesions, while expanding, has yet to yield instrumentation superior to other modalities. Consequently, much attention focuses on the efficacy of the perioperative use of surgical adjuvants to further improve operative outcome. While most would concur that adjuvants do not represent a replacement for inferior skills, they have the potential to optimize the postoperative status of the pelvis.

As illustrated in many of the presentations, the future represents the rapid dawning of a better understanding of the factors responsible for postoperative adhesion development. The increased attention and resources being utilized to address these important issues allow identification of pathways to win the war against adhesions and the multitude of problems they cause.

Michael P. Diamond
Gere S. diZerega
Cary B. Linsky
Robert L. Reid

Gynecologic Surgery and Adhesion Prevention, pages 1–18

THE CAUSE AND PREVENTION OF POSTSURGICAL ADHESIONS: A CONTEMPORARY UPDATE

Gere S. diZerega, M.D.
Professor of Obstetrics and Gynecology
Livingston Reproductive Biology Laboratory
Department of Obstetrics and Gynecology
University of Southern California School of Medicine
Los Angeles County-University of Southern California Medical Center
1321 North Mission Road
Los Angeles, California 90033

Peritoneum is the most extensive serous membrane in the body. The surface area of the peritoneum is generally equal to that of the skin ranging from 8,800-12,000 cm^2 for adults (177 cm^2/kg body weight) to 475-1,400 cm^2 for infants and children (383 cm^2/kg body weight). It is composed of mesothelial cells which form a continuous layer resting upon loose mesenchymal connective tissue, a basal lamina, and basement membrane which is attached to the abdominal wall and viscera by areolar tissue (subserous fascia) (diZerega and Rodgers, 1992). The apical surface of the mesothelial cells contains an abundance of long microvilli which increase the functional surface area of the peritoneum for both absorption and secretion. The peritoneum is well supplied with blood vessels and lymphatics which give rise to a rich capillary network. It serves to minimize friction facilitating free movement between abdominal viscera, resists or localizes infection, and stores fat especially in the greater omentum.

PERITONEAL RE-EPITHELIALIZATION

General agreement exists between investigators that regeneration of mesothelium layer occurs within 5-8 days for all peritoneal surfaces. Ellis et al. (1965) and Hubbard (1967) reported that healing occurs in 5-6 days in the case of parietal peritoneum. Glucksman (1966) reports that the visceral mesothelium covering the terminal ileum heals in 5 days, while Eskeland (1966a) demonstrated that regeneration of the mesothelial layer of parietal peritoneum is complete by 8 days. Raftery confirmed the findings of Eskeland (1966a) that parietal peritoneum of the rat is healed within 8 days.

Raftery (1973a) studied the regeneration of parietal and visceral peritoneum using scanning electron microscopy. Twelve hours after injury, numerous polymorphonuclear leukocytes (PMNs) were seen intangled in fibrin strands. At 24-36 hrs after wounding the number of cells in the superficial part of the wound was greatly increased; most of the increase in cell number was due to infiltration by macrophages. At 2 days most of the wound surface was covered with a single layer of macrophages supported by a fibrin scaffold. The cells on the wound surface at 3 days were similar to primitive mesenchymal cells. At 4 days cells resembling primitive mesenchymal cells or proliferating fibroblasts on the wound surface were in contact with one another. In some areas healing appeared complete at 5 days since a single layer of mesothelial cells was present on the wound surface in both parietal and visceral peritoneum. By the fifth day after injury there were essentially no differences between parietal and visceral peritoneal repair. On the surface of wounds of both the parietal visceral peritoneum, cells appeared to be uniform resembling proliferating fibroblasts connected by tight junctions. Seven days after injury, continuous layers of mesothelial cells cover the surface of both the visceral and parietal peritoneum. By the eighth day, the basement membrane beneath the mesothelial cells of both types of peritoneum is continuous. Visceral peritoneum appears to differ little in its healing properties from the parietal peritoneum.

Neonate

Raftery (1973b) described the healing of visceral and parietal peritoneum in the immature rat at various times after standardized surgical injury to the liver capsule and parietal peritoneum. Although the wounds looked hemorrhagic and uneven 24 hours after injury, they were smooth and glistening at 3 days, and usually indistinguishable from the normal surrounding parietal peritoneum at 5 days. The cellular changes which accompanied these gross morphological changes were the same as those described for the adult except that mesothelial regeneration occurred more rapidly. By 5 days the number of macrophages diminished leaving only fibroblasts. These fibroblasts came together to form the new mesothelium by 7 days. In the case of visceral peritoneum, mesothelial regeneration was complete by 5 days. Again, there was no substantive difference in the rate of healing between visceral and parietal peritoneal defects.

MORPHOGENESIS OF ADHESION FORMATION

The process of adhesion formation is the same for visceral and parietal peritoneum. The initiation of adhesion formation begins with a fibrin matrix which typically occurs during coagulation. This matrix is gradually replaced by vascular granulation tissue containing macrophages, fibroblasts and giant cells. The clots are slow to achieve complete organization. In the process, they consist of erythrocytes separated by strands or condensed masses of fibrin which are covered with two or three layers of flattened cells and contain a patchy infiltrate of mononuclear cells. Eventually the adhesion matures into a fibrous band which is often covered by mesothelium and contains blood vessels and connective tissue fibers, including elastin.

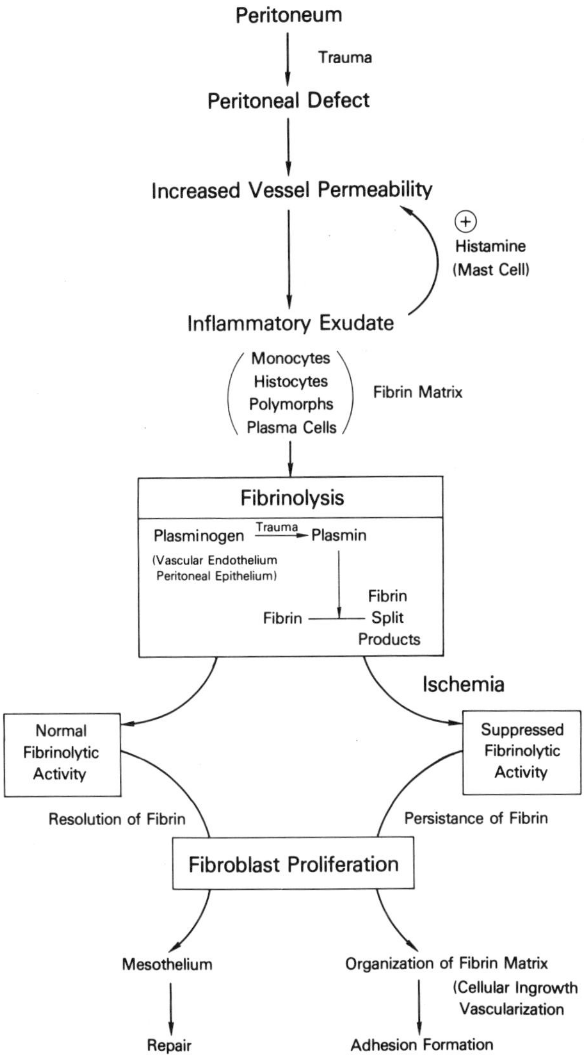

Figure 1
Summary of normal tissue repair and adhesion formation following surgical trauma. After trauma to the peritoneum, there is increased vascular permeability, mediated by histamine, which produces an inflammatory exudate and formation of fibrin matrix. As with other parts of the body, this fibrin matrix is normally removed by fibrinolysis.

Under normal conditions, where fibrinolytic activity is allowed to occur, fibroblast proliferation results in remesothelialization. However, under the ischemic conditions present in surgical trauma, fibrinolytic activity is suppressed and fibrin is allowed to persist. Once the fibrin bands are infiltrated with fibroblasts, they become organized into adhesions. (From Montz et al., 1987)

Milligan and Raftery described the histological and morphological features of postsurgical adhesion formation in rats using light and electron microscopic techniques (1974). They compared adhesions arising from the liver, cecum and ileal-cecal junction using both peritoneal abrasion and stripping techniques to create petechial bleeding or a clear, well demarcated peritoneal defect. Rats were sacrificed 7 or 14 days as well as 1 or 2 months after the initial trauma. No differences were noted in the formation of adhesions in these different areas.

At day 1-3 the adhesion was characterized by a variety of cellular elements encased in a fibrin matrix. The cells were primarily PMNs but also included macrophages, eosinophils, red blood cells (RBC) and tissue debris as well as necrotic cells presumably desquamated from the peritoneal injury. By 4 days macrophages were the predominant leukocyte in the fibrin mesh which was associated with a few fibroblasts. In contrast many fibroblasts were lying together forming a syncytium. Distinct bundles of collagen were evident as were scattered foreign body granulomas. At 7 days collagen and fibroblasts were the predominant components of the adhesion. However, small vascular channels containing endothelial cells were present. Over the next 2 weeks to 2 months cellularity of the adhesion was replaced almost entirely by collagen fibrils associated with macrophages.

Animal Models: Adhesion Induction

To obtain peritoneal adhesions in animals, it is necessary to inflict severe damage usually involving two adjacent surfaces or to use artificial methods (see reviews: Richardson, 1911; Boys, 1942; Connolly and Smith, 1960). The following are descriptions of injuries used to induce adhesion formation in standard animal models.

1. Mechanical injury: crushing the bowel, (Thomas et al., 1950; Spagna et al., 1961; Choate et al., 1964; Grosz et al., 1966; Perriard et al., 1966; Swolin, 1966); stripping or scrubbing away the outer layers from long segments of bowel wall (Pope, 1914; Warren, 1928; Lacey, 1930; Trusler, 1931; Thomas et al., 1950; Hubay et al., 1953; de Sanctis et al., 1955; Gustavsson et al., 1955).

2. Ischemia: dividing major vessels to loops of intestine, (Ellis, 1963; James et al., 1965).

3. Introduction of foreign material: talcum (German, 1943; Seelig et al., 1943; Zachariae, 1954; Luttwak et al., 1957; Myllärniemi et al., 1966; Myllärniemi, 1967 colloidal silica, Green et al., 1970; Schade et al., 1968); gauze sponges (Adams, 1913; Donaldson, 1938; Lehman et al., 1940); toxic chemicals (Warren, 1928; Lacey, 1930; Heinz, 1900; Chandy, 1950); bacteria (Adams, 1913; Mion et al., 1965); feces (Jackson, 1958).

Table 1

Incidence of Adhesions at Initial Surgery and Follow-up Laparoscopy[a]

Tissue	Adhesion Rate			
	Initial Surgery[b]		Follow-up Laparoscopy[c]	
	No.	%	No.	%
Ovaries	303/387	78%	207/376	55%
Fimbria	244/384	64%	135/372	36%
Cul-de-sac	87/208	42%	42/208	20%
Omentum	32/208	15%	39/208	19%
Colon	63/208	14%	30/204	15%
Small intestine	30/208	14%	30/208	14%
Pelvic sidewall	124/208	60%	84/208	40%

[a] Adapted from Diamond et al. (1987).
[b] Initial surgery performed using CO_2 laser + 35% Dextran 70 or non-laser surgical technique with or without Dextran. Results are pooled over three initial surgical procedure groups.
[c] Within 12 weeks of initial surgery.

Table 2

Pelvic Adhesions Noted at Second-Look Laparoscopy

	Time from Initial Procedure	Total No. of Patients	Total No. with Adhesions	% with Adhesions
Diamond (32)	1 Wk - 12 Wk	106	91	86
DeCherney and Mezer (34)	4 Wk - 16 Wk	20	15	75
	1Yr - 3 Yr	41	31	76
Surrey and Friedman (148)	6 Wk - 8 Wk	31	22	71
	≥ 6 Mo	6	5	83
Pittaway (155)	4 Wk - 6 Wk	23	23	100
Trimbos-Kemper (60)	8 Days	188	104	55
Daniell and Pittaway (153)	4 Wk - 6 Wk	25	24	96

DIAMOND MP. IN: SCIARRA JW, ED. GYNECOLOGY AND OBSTETRICS. VOL 5. PHILADELPHIA, PA: HARPER & ROW; CHP 61, Pg.5, 1988.

Fibrin

Fibrinous exudate is a necessary precursor for fibrous adhesions. Highly mobile intraperitoneal structures will not permanently adhere to each other unless held in continuous, close apposition until fibroblast invasion leads to collagen deposition beginning on the third postoperative day. Thus, the crucial consideration is the factor which determines whether the fibrinous adhesion is absorbed, or persists and is organized (Ellis, 1971; Ellis, 1983). Fibrin provides the initial bridge between two surfaces; when the bridge is made of fibrin only, it is amenable to lysis by fibrinolytic mechanisms; but when it contains cellular elements (erythrocytes, leukocytes, platelets etc.) within the fibrin it will likely undergo organization into an adhesion. Under these experimental conditions (1) desquamation of mesothelial cells appears to be the critical event in adhesion formation and (2) adhesions apparently develop only when 2 denuded surfaces are involved.

PREDISPOSING FACTORS

Sex

There does not appear to be a sex bias in the development of postoperative adhesions. Weibel & Majno (1973) reported a slightly higher frequency of adhesions among male patients. After excluding adhesions resulting from gynecologic procedures, Raf (1969) reported that the incidence of intraperitoneal adhesions was 47% in male patients and 53% in female patients.

Anatomical Site

The omentum is particularly susceptible to adhesion formation. In Weibel and Majno's studies (1973), the omentum was involved in 92% of postoperative adhesions. The omentum was also the predominant organ involved in "spontaneous" adhesions (i.e., those with no prior history of surgery); 100% of the 126 spontaneous adhesions examined by Weibel and Majno involved the omentum. With the exception of the omentum, the internal organs involved in postoperative adhesions may vary as a function of the surgical procedure. The small intestine was involved in 21% of the adhesions present after appendectomy but in only 6% of those formed following gynecologic laparotomy; 47% and 19% of adhesions which form after appendectomy and gynecologic laparotomy, respectively, involve the colon (Turunen, 1933). The ovary is the most common site for adhesions to form after reconstructive surgery of the female pelvis (Table 1, Adhesion Study Group, 1983; Interceed (TC7) Adhesion Barrier Study Group, 1989; Diamond et al., 1987). Ovarian adhesions were found at second-look laparoscopy in over 90% of cases after ovarian surgery (Pittaway et al., 1985).

PREVENTION OF ADHESION FORMATION

While careful attention to surgical techniques reduces the likelihood of adhesion formation, these efforts by themselves are unable to prevent adhesion formation (Table 2). Thus, adjuvant therapy is needed for adhesion free healing. There is an extensive literature describing agents tried in the prevention of postoperative adhesion formation. Certainly the most promising medicament for future investigation is the non-steroidal anti-inflammatory drug group (Table 3). In vitro studies show that these drugs inhibit adhesion formation through suppression of plasminogen activator inhibitor which enhances plasminogen activator activity and, as a result, fibrinolysis (Rodgers et al., 1990, 1992). The systemic administration of pharmacologic agents to prevent formation of postsurgical adhesions in clinical and animal studies has not met with the success in vitro studies predicted. Systemic administration of medicaments requires adequate blood supply to the site of adhesion formation so that sufficient tissue levels are available to achieve pharmacological effects. The blood supply is often removed from surgical sites during the procedure. These ischemic areas are common sites for adhesion formation. Accordingly, one of the major challenges to the pharmacotherapy of adhesion prevention is development of appropriate delivery systems. To date, no single therapeutic approach has proven universally effective in preventing formation of postoperative adhesions.

Intraperitoneal Solutions As Barriers

Animal studies show that mechanical barriers can prevent adhesion formation by limiting tissue apposition during the initial phases of peritoneal repair (Soules et al., 1982). Barriers for adhesion prevention are available in both liquid and solid preparations. Many years ago, Kajihara reported that a constituent of the extracellular matrix, chondroitin sulfate, is useful in this regard (Kajihara, 1960). More recently, Elkins (1984a,b) and Fredericks et al. (1986) showed that carboxymethyl cellulose prevented the formation of adhesions in animal models. Thus, chondroitin sulfate and carboxymethyl cellulose both show promise as liquid barriers to adhesion formation. However, their clinical utility awaits the scrutiny of toxicity studies and clinical trials.

Dextran is a water-soluble polymer of glucose that was originally developed as a plasma expander. Of all the intraperitoneal agents evaluated for adhesion prevention it has received the most attention. Although dextran can be manufactured in a variety of molecular weights, most of the research focused on 32% dextran 70 (Hyskon, Pharmacia; molecular weight 70,000). In the initial clinical trial, performed in the United States, 32% dextran 70 was found to have limited benefit in reducing adhesion formation (Adhesion Study Group, 1983). This was not confirmed in a follow up study performed in Sweden using the same protocol (Larsson et al., 1985) and in a subsequent study of infertility patients performed in Australia (Jansen, 1985).

Oelsner et al. (1987) compared these liquid barriers in an animal model and found chondroitin sulfate superior to both carboxymethyl cellulose or Hyskon in preventing postsurgical adhesions. However, by comparing the regimens in a standardized rat model, Graebe et al. found carboxymethyl cellulose as effective as chondroitin sulfate and significantly better than Hyskon, in preventing adhesions (Graebe et al., 1989).

Barriers

Ideally, a physical barrier for adhesion prevention should be completely absorbable and nonreactive; furthermore, it should stay in place within the body without the use of sutures or staples. A polytetrafluoroethylene barrier (Gore-Tex) (Boyers et al., 1988) was shown to reduce the formation of post surgical adhesions in a rabbit uterine horn model. However, this result was not confirmed in a similar animal study (Goldberg et al., 1987). Gore-Tex has many drawbacks as a clinically useful barrier: in must be sutured in place, it is nonabsorbable, and cannot expand when used to cover the uterus.

Table 3
Animal Studies Performed to Assess the Efficacy of Nonsteroidal Antiinflammatory Drugs as Adjuvents to Prevent Formation of Postsurgical Adhesions

Author	Animal model	Iburprofen dosage[a]	Results	Reference
Siegler et al.	Rabbit uterine horn transection with unilateral reanastomosis and contralateral cautery	7mg/kg three times daily x 2 days, IV	5/9 control--dense adhesions 7/7 treated--filmy adhesions	Fertil Steril 34:46, 1980
Bateman et al.	Rabbit uterine horn linear incisions with repair and contralateral abrasion	10mg/kg three times daily x 4 days, IV or 10 mg/kg, IP	Mean adhesion score in control 0.9; IV, 0.2; IP, 0.5	Surg Forum 32:603, 1981
Holtz	Rabbit uterine horn crush and abrasion with lysis of adhesions 2 weeks later	12.5 mg/kg two times daily x 3 days, IM	No significant reduction in reformation	Fertil Steril 37:582, 1982
Bateman et al.	Rabbit uterine horn crush and abrasion	10 mg/kg three times daily 4 days, IV	Significant reduction	Fertil Steril 38:107, 1982
O'Brien et al.	Oophorectomy and contralateral salpingo-oophorectomy in ewes	5 mg/kg three times daily x 2 days, IM	No significant reduction	Obstet Gynecol 60:373, 1982
Nishimura et al.	Rabbit uterine horn abrasion, crushing or devascularization	70 mg/kg x 2, IM or 70 mg/kg four times	No reduction with 2 doses; significant with 5 doses	J Surg Res 34:219, 1983
Luciano et al.	Rat uterine horn transection with unilateral reanastomosis and contralateral cautery	12.5 mg/kg three times daily x 2 days, IP	No significant reduction	Am J Obst Gyn 146:88, 1983

[a]IV, intravenous; IP, intraperitoneal; IM, intramuscular.

Oxidized regenerated cellulose (ORC) appears to satisfy the criteria of an ideal barrier. This material is completely absorbable and is minimally reactive. ORC maintains its position within the peritoneum without the use of sutures when residual peritoneal fluid is minimized. Initial studies with ORC evaluated the use of Surgicel, an absorbable material that is used extensively for hemostasis. Some studies in animal models show that Surgicel it is able to reduce the severity and/or incidence of adhesion formation. A significant reduction in adhesion formation was demonstrated in the rat cecal model (Larsson et al., 1978), rat multiple peritoneal trauma and ischemic peritoneal models (Raferty, 1980); rabbit uterine horn model (Galan et al., 1983; Nishimura et al., 1983; Shimanuki et al., 1987) and rabbit bowel reanastomosis model (Shimanuki and Nishimura, 1987).

However, not all studies demonstrated efficacy of Surgicel in preventing adhesions.

Schroder (Schroder et al., 1982) and Yemini (Yemini et al., 1984) evaluated Surgicel among other modalities and failed to demonstrate a reduction in cecal adhesions in rats. Soules et al. (1982) found that Surgicel offered no benefit after a standardized cut or scrape of the rabbit uterine horn. Hixson et al. (1986) studied the ability of Surgicel to prevent postsurgical adhesions to the fimbria and ovaries; Surgicel did not reduce adnexal adhesions.

Interceed

Recently, a modification of Surgicel was found to be more effective in preventing adhesion formation in the rabbit (Linsky et al., 1987; Diamond et al., 1987). This new material (Interceed) is also made of oxidized regenerated cellulose. The difference is that the knitted pattern was changed so that Interceed has a longer intraperitoneal residence time than Surgicel. A significant reduction in adhesion formation was observed following use of Interceed after uterine or peritoneal sidewall trauma in the rabbit (Diamond et al., 1987; Linksy et al., 1987; 1988). In October 1989 Interceed received approval by the Food and Drug Administration as the first adjuvant indicated for the reduction of postsurgical adhesions.

CLINICAL EVALUATIONS

North American Study

A prospective, multicenter, randomized evaluation of Interceed was conducted to assess clinical efficacy (Interceed (TC7) Adhesion Barrier Study Group, 1989; Malinak, 1990). Infertility patients (n=134) in 13 investigational centers underwent lysis of bilateral pelvic sidewall adhesions. Following adhesiolysis, the area of the deperitonealized surface was measured. Interceed was applied in an amount sufficient to completely cover deperitonealized surfaces on the sidewall; the contralateral sidewall was left uncovered, thereby serving as control. A second-look laparoscopy was performed between 10 days and 14 weeks after the laparotomy. Interceed barrier was found to significantly reduce the incidence (Table 4), extent and severity of postoperative adhesions. Interceed also significantly reduced adhesion formation between ovaries and peritoneal sidewall. In a matched-sidewall comparison, Interceed was four times more effective than surgery alone in preventing adhesion reformation (Table 5, 46 vs 10).

Japanese Study

Clinical efficacy shown in the initial study with Interceed was recently confirmed by a multicenter study performed in Japan (Sekiba et al., 1991; Table 4; Figure 3). Sixty-three infertility patients in 12 investigational centers participated in a prospective, randomized study. All patients had both tubes and ovaries as well as bilateral pelvic sidewall adhesions. After completion of all operative procedures including lysis of adhesions, a sealed envelope was opened which identified the pelvic sidewall to be

Table 4

Adhesions Present (+) or Absent (-) on Sidewall of Women at Second-Look Laparoscopy

Interceed Treated	Absent	Present	Absent	Present	
Control Sidewall	Present	Absent	Absent	Present	
North American Study (Malinak et al., 1991)	34%	7%	16%	41%	n=134
Japanese Study (Sekiba et al., 1991)	39%	4%	19%	36%	n=63
Combined	36%	6%	17%	40%	n=197

Table 5

Matched Pair Comparison of Treatment Effect Sidewalls With No Adhesions

Study	Interceed	Control	Interceed Benefit
North American (Malinak et al., 1991)	46 (82%)	10 (17%)	4.6x
Japanese (Sekiba et al., 1991)	25 (89%)	3 (10%)	8.3x
Combined	71 (84%)	13 (15%)	5.5x

covered with Interceed. The incidence and extent of adhesion reformation along the pelvic sidewalls were determined at second-look laparoscopy performed between 10 days and 14 weeks after laparotomy. At laparoscopy, 37 of 63 (59%) Interceed-treated sidewalls and 15 of 63 (23%) control sidewalls did not contain adhesions. In a matched-sidewall comparison, Interceed was 8 times more effective than surgery alone (control) in preventing adhesion reformation (Table 5, 25 versus 3). Interceed-treated sidewalls had significantly less area involved with adhesions compared with the control sidewall (Figure 3). The deperitonealized areas (DAs) for all sidewalls were divided into three groups (group I: DA<100mm^2, n=72; group II: 100mm^2≤DA<1000mm^2, n=95; group III: 1000mm^2≤DA, n=38). All Interceed (TC7) treated groups had significantly less area involved with adhesions than the control sidewalls at laparoscopy.

Mechanism of Adhesion Prevention

Larsson suggested that oxidized regenerated cellulose prevents adhesion formation by its transformation into a gelatinous mass that covers the damaged peritoneum and thereby protects it from involvement in adhesion formation (Larsson et al., 1978). This gelatinous "cocoon" seems to provide a protective coating over healing tissue during the initial postoperative interval (Linksy et al., 1987; Diamond et al., 1987). During this time, re-epithelialization of damaged peritoneal surfaces is completed (7-10 days, diZerega and Rodgers, 1992).

Study Comparisons

Interceed was 8 times (Japanese Study) and 4 times (North American Study) more effective than state-of-the-art surgery alone in preventing the reformation of adhesions when there was a difference between the sidewalls in the same patient (Table 5). Comparison of differences in results of the North American and Japanese studies are instructive for developing the best technique for Interceed application. In the North American study an effort was made to carefully "picture frame" the area of surgical injury with Interceed. Only the area of injury was covered with no room for overlap of the perimeter. At second-look laparoscopy adhesions found near or in the sidewall study site were difficult to evaluate. In order to eliminate this ambiguity a larger piece of Interceed was used in the Japanese study. Interceed extended beyond the perimeter of the surgical injury leaving a 3-5 mm overlap. This Interceed border beyond the surgical site provides a more effective barrier between peri-surgical areas of inflammation and adjacent tissues.

The Japanese investigators evaluated photographs made at the time of initial laparotomy in the North American Study. In some cases when adhesions formed in the Interceed treated site, as determined at second-look laparoscopy, the Interceed was noted to have turned dark brown or even black after application at laparotomy. This contamination of the barrier by blood contributed to adhesion reformation. Fibrin from blood impregnated the Interceed barrier and reduced its ability to prevent adhesions. As a result, the Japanese investigators were careful to remove any Interceed that turned brown or black. In those cases they reestablished sufficient hemostasis so that a new piece of Interceed could be applied over the surgical site without contamination by blood. Sometimes this required additional suturing of the tissue around the bleeding site or futher coagulation. If Interceed turns black its ability to prevent adhesions is compromised. Recent evidence suggests that local application of thrombin over the oozing site achieves adequate hemostasis for Interceed application (Wiseman et al., 1991).

The third technical point for Interceed use I learned performing laparoscopic surgery. After removal of an ovarian cyst I wrapped the ovary with Interceed. As the patient was taken out of Trendelenburg position the patient's pelvis moved into a gravitationally-dependent position. Peritoneal fluid from under the diaphragm and in the colonic gutters entered the pelvis and washed the Interceed off of the ovary. Now I place the patient in reverse Trendelenburg position at the end of surgery (both laparotomy and laparoscopy). In reverse Trendelenburg position the peritoneal fluid can be effectively aspirated from the cul-de-sac which is the most gravitationally dependent area. Thereafter the patient is returned to a position in which the specific site(s) for Interceed application can best be accessed.

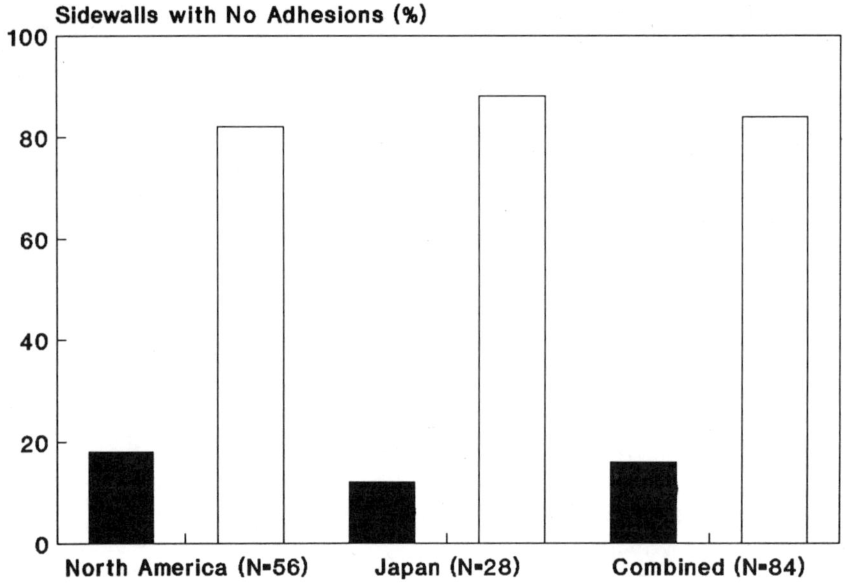

Figure 2
Interceed was found to significantly reduce adhesion reformation to the pelvic side wall compared to state-of-the-art surgery alone (open bar) as determined by multicenter clinical studies in North America (Malinak, 1991) and Japan (Sekiba et al., 1991).

Perspective

Should Interceed be used after every case of gynecological surgery? - No. Many cases do not allow for sufficient hemostasis or adequate removal of peritoneal fluid. The technology is limited. However, as a first step towards effective adhesion prevention, Interceed has made real progress. The two large clinical data sets now available show that sufficient attention to the details of application will lead to a real reduction in the formation of postsurgical adhesions.

As a first step, these studies are a landmark in adhesion prevention. However, as clinicians we need to know if clinical benefit can be derived from Interceed use. Studies of "clinical efficacy" have only assesed the presence or absence of adhesions and not the clinical benefits of adhesion prevention per se. Demonstration of clinical benefit requires large studies with prolonged follow-up time which allow for delineation of the multifactorial co-variants of clinical response to treatment. Perhaps these types of "second generation" studies will be employed to directly address the clinical benefit of this promising new technology.

REFERENCES

Adams JE (1913): Peritoneal adhesions (an experimental study). Lancet 1:663-668.

Adhesion Study Group (1983): Reduction of postoperative pelvic adhesions with intraperitoneal 32% dextran 70: a prospective, randomized clinical trial. Fertil Steril 40:612-619.

Bloom W, Fawcett DW (1975): "A Textbook of Histology" (9th Edition). PA: Saunders, pp 186-188.

Boyers SP, Diamond MP, DeCherney AH (1988): Reduction of postoperative pelvic adhesions in the rabbit with Gore-Tex surgical membrane. Fertil Steril 49:1066-1070.

Boys F (1942): The prophylaxis of peritoneal adhesions: a review of the literature. Surgery 11:118-168.

Bridges JB, Whitting HW (1964): Parietal peritoneal healing in the rat. J Path Bact 87:123-130.

Chandy J (1950): Use of heparin in the prevention of peritoneal adhesions. Arch Surg 60:1151-1153.

Choate WH, Just-Viera JO, Yaeger GH (1964): Prevention of experimental peritoneal adhesions by dextran. Arch Surg 88:249-254.

Connolly JE, Smith JW (1960): The prevention and treatment of intestinal adhesions. Int Abstr Surgery 110:417-431.

Daniell JF, Pittaway DE (1983): Short-interval second-look laparoscopy after infertility surgery: a preliminary report. J Reprod Med 28:281-283.

de Sanctis AL, Schatten WE, Weckesser EC (1955): Effect of hydrocortisone in the prevention of intraperitoneal adhesions. Arch Surg 71:523-530.

DeCherney AH, Mezer HC (1984): The nature of posttuboplasty pelvic adhesions as determined by early and late laparoscopy. Fertil Steril 41:643-646.

Diamond MP, Linsky CB, Cunningham T, Constantine B, diZerega GS, DeCherney AH (1987): A model for sidewall adhesions in the rabbit: reduction by an absorbable barrier. Microsurg 8:197-200.

Diamond MP, Daniell JF, Feste J, Surrey MW, McLaughin DS, Friedman S, Vaughn WK, Martin DC (1987): Adhesion formation and de novo adhesion formation after reproductive pelvic surgery. Fertil Steril 47:864-866.

Diamond MP, DeCherney AH (1987): Pathogenesis of adhesion formation/ reformation: application to reproductive pelvic surgery. Microsurgery 8:103-107.

diZerega GS (1990): The peritoneum and its response to surgical injury. In diZerega GS, Malinak LR, Diamond MP, Linsky CB (eds): "Treatment of Post Surgical Adhesions." (Progress in Clinical and Biological Research, Vol 358). New York: Wiley-Liss, Inc., pp 1-11.

diZerega GS, Rodgers KE (1992): "The Peritoneum" (1st ed.). New York: Springer Verlag.

Donaldson JK (1938): Abdominal adhesions and the use of papain: a discussion and an experimental study. Arch Surg 36:20-27.

Elkins TE, Bury RJ, Ritter JL, Ling FW, Ahokas RA, Homsey CA, Malinak LR (1984a): Adhesion prevention by solutions of sodium carboxymethylcellulose in the rat. I. Fertil Steril 41:926-928.

Elkins TE, Ling FW, Ahokas RA Abdella TN, Homsey CA, Malinak LR (1984b): Adhesion prevention by solutions of sodium carboxymethylcellulose in the rat.II. Fertil Steril 41:929-932.

Ellis H (1963): The aetiology of post-operative abdominal adhesions: an experimental study. Brit J Surg 50:10-16.

Ellis H, Harrison W, Hugh TB (1965): The healing of peritoneum under normal and pathological conditions. Brit J Surg 52:471-476.

Ellis H (1971): The cause and prevention of postoperative intraperitoneal adhesions. Surg Gynecol Obstet 133:497-511.

Ellis H (1983): Prevention and treatment of adhesions. Infect Surg 803-818.

Eskeland G, Kjærheim Å (1966a): Regeneration of parietal peritoneum in rats. I. A light microscopical study. Acta Pathol Microbiol Scandinav 68:353-378.

Esperanza MJ, Collins DL (1966): Peritoneal dialysis efficiency in relation to body weight. J Ped Surg 1:162-169.

Fredericks CM, Kotry I, Holtz G, Askalani AH, Serour GI (1986): Adhesion prevention in the rabbit with sodium carboxymethylcellulose solutions. Am J Obstet Gynecol 155:667-670.

Galan N, Leader A, Malkinson T, Taylor PJ (1983): Adhesion prophylaxis in rabbits with Surgicel and two absorbable microsurgical sutures. J Reprod Med 28:662-664.

German WMCK (1943): Dusting powder granulomas following surgery. Surg Gynec Obstet 76:501-507.

Glucksman D (1966): Serosal integrity and intestinal adhesions. Surgery 60:1009-1011.

Goldberg JM, Toledo AA, Mitchell DE (1987): An evaluation of the Gore-Tex surgical membrane for the prevention of postoperative peritoneal adhesions. Obstet Gynecol 70:846-848.

Graebe RA, Oelsner G, Cornelison TL, Pan S-B, Haseltine FP, DeCherney AH (1989): An animal study of different treatments to prevent postoperative pelivc adhesions. Microsurgery 10:53-55.

Green N, French S, Fingerhut A (1970): Radiation inhibition of peritoneal adhesions: an experimental study. Proc Soc Exp Biol Med 133:544-550.

Grosz C, Aka E, Zimmer J, Alterwein R (1966): The effect of intraperitoneal fluids on the prevention of experimental adhesions. Surgery 60:1232-1234.

Gustavsson E, Blombäck B, Blombäck M, Wallen P (1955): Plasmin in the prevention of adhesions: preliminary report. Acta Chir Scand 109:327-333.

Heinz Ueber die Herkunft des (1900): Fibrins und die Enstehung von Verwachsuger bie acutes adhäsiver Entzündung seröser Haute. Virchow Arch [Path Anat] 160:365-377.

Hixson C, Swanson LA, Friedman CI (1986): Oxidized cellulose for preventing adnexal adhesions. J Reprod Med 31:58-60.

Hubay CA, Weckesser EC, Holden WD (1953): The effect of cortisone on the prevention of peritoneal adhesions. Surg Gynec Obstet 96:65-70.

Hubbard TB, Khan MZ, Carag VR, Albites VE, Hricko GM (1967): The pathology of peritoneal repair: its relation to the formation of adhesions. Ann Surg 165:908-916.

Interceed(TC7) Adhesion Barrier Study Group (1989): Prevention of postsurgical adhesions by Interceed(TC7), an absorbable adhesion barrier: a prospective, randomized multicenter clinical study. Fertil Steril 51:933-938.

Jackson BB (1958): Observations on intraperitoneal adhesions, an experimental study. Surgery 44:507-518.

James DCO, Ellis H, Hugh TB (1965): The effect of streptokinase on experimental intraperitoneal adhesion fromation. J Path Bact 90:279-287.

Jansen RPS (1985): Failure of intraperitoneal adjuncts to improve the outcome of pelvic operations in young women. Am J Obstet Gynecol 153:363-371.

Johnson FR, Whitting HW (1962): Repair of parietal peritoneum. Brit J Surg 49:653-660.

Kajihara Y (1960): The use of chondroitin sulfuric acid for the prevention of peritoneal adhesions. J Kurume Med Assoc 23:4641-4649.

Lacey JT (1930): The prevention of peritoneal adhesions by amniotic fluid. Ann Surg 92:281-293.

Larsson B, Nisell H, Granberg I (1978): Surgicel - an absorbable hemostatic material - in prevention of peritoneal adhesions in rats. Acta Chir Scand 144:375-378.

Larsson B, Lalos O, Marsk L, Tronstad SE, Bygdeman M, Pehrson S, Joelson I (1985): Effect of intraperitoneal instillation of 32% dextran 70 on postoperative adhesion formation after tubal surgery. Acta Obstet Gynecol Scand 64:437-441.

Lehman EP, Boys F (1940): The prevention of peritoneal adhesions with heparin: an experimental study. Ann Surg 111:427-435.

Linsky CB, Diamond MP, Cunningham T, Constantine B, DeCherney AH, diZerega GS (1987): Adhesion reduction in the rabbit uterine horn model using an absorbable barrier, TC-7. J Reprod Med 32:17-20.

Linsky CB, Diamond MP, Cunningham, T, DeCherney AH, diZerega GS (1988): Effect of blood on the efficacy of barrier adhesion reduction in the rabbit uterine horn model. Infertility 11:273-280.

Luttwak EM, Behar AJ, Saltz NJ (1957): Effect of fibrinolytic agents and corticosteroid hormones on peritoneal adhesions: a comparative experimental study. Arch Surg 75:96-101.

Malinak LR (1990): Interceed (TC7) as an adjuvant for adhesion reduction: clinical studies. In diZerega GS, Malinak LR, Diamond M, Linsky C (eds): "Treatment of Postoperative Surgical Adhesion." New York: Wiley-Liss, pp 193-206.

Milligan DW, Raftery AT (1974): Observations on the pathogenesis of peritoneal adhesions: a light and electron microscopical study. Br J Surg 61:274-280.

Mion CM, Boen ST (1965): Analysis of factors responsible for the formation of adhesions during chronic peritoneal dialysis. Am J Med Sci 250:675-679.

Montz FJ, Shimanuki T, diZerega GS (1987): Postsurgical mesothelial re-epithelialization. In DeCherney AH, Polan ML (eds): "Reproductive Surgery." Chicago: Year Book Medical Publishers, Inc., pp 31-47.

Myllärniemi H, Frilander M, Turunen M, Saxén L (1966): The effect of glove powders and their constituents on adhesion and granuloma formation in the abdominal cavity of the rabbit. Acta Chir Scand 131:312-318.

Myllärniemi H (1967): Foreign material adhesion formation after abdominal surgery: a clinical and experimental study. Acta Chir Scand 377:1-48.

Nishimura K, Nakamura RM, diZerega GS (1983): Biochemical evaluation of postsurgical wound repair: prevention of intraperitoneal adhesion formation with ibuprofen. J Surg Res 34:219-226.

Oelsner G, Graebe RA, Pan S-B, Haseltine FP, Barnea ER, Fakih H, DeCherney AH (1987): Chondroitin sulphate. A new intraperitoneal treatment for postoperative adhesion prevention in the rabbit. J Reprod Med 32:812-814.

Perriard M, Mirkovitch V (1966): L'effet du diméthyloplysiloxane sur la prévention d'adhérences abdominals chez le rat. Helv Chir Acta 33:536-540.

Pittaway DE, Daniell JF, Maxson WS (1985): Ovarian surgery in an infertility patient as an indicator for a short-interval second-look laparoscopy: A preliminary report. Fertil Steril 44:611-614.

Pope S (1914): The use of citrate solutions in the prevention of peritoneal adhesions. Ann Surg 59:101-106.

Raf LE (1969): Causes of abdominal adhesions in cases of intestinal obstruction. Acta Chir Scand 135:73-76.

Raftery AT (1973a): Regeneration of parietal and visceral peritoneum: an electron microscopical study. J Anat 115:375-392.

Raftery AT (1973b): Regeneration of parietal and visceral peritoneum. A light microscopical study. Brit J Surg 60:293-299.

Raftery AT (1980): Absorbable haemostatic materials and intraperitoneal adhesion formation. Brit J Surg 67:57-58.

Raftery AT (1981): Effect of peritoneal trauma on peritoneal fibrinolytic activity and intraperitoneal adhesion formation. An experimental study in the rat. Eur Surg Res 13:397-401.

Richardson EH (1911): Studies on peritoneal adhesions: with a contribution to the treatment of denuded surfaces. Amer Surg 54:758-797.

Rodgers KE (1990): Non steroidal anti-inflammatory drugs (NSAIDs) in the treatment of postsurgical adhesions. In diZerega GS, Malinak LR, Diamond MD, Linsky C (eds): "Treatment of Postsurgical Adhesions." (Progress in Clinical and Biological Research, Vol 358). New York: Wiley-Liss, pp 119-130.

Rodgers K, Ellefson D, Girgis W, diZerega GS (1992): Protease and protease inhibitor secretion following in vitro exposure to tolmetin. Agents and Actions (in review).

Schade DS, Williamson JR (1968): The pathogenesis of peritoneal adhesions: an ultrastructural study. Ann Surg 167:500-510.

Schroder M, Willumsen H, Hart Hansen JP, Hart Hansen O (1982): Peritoneal adhesion formation after the use of oxidized cellulose (Surgicel) and gelatin sponge (Spongostan) in rats. Acta Chir Scand

148:595-596.

Seelig MG, Verda DJ, Kidd FH (1943): The talcum powder problem in surgery and its solution. J Am Med Assoc 23:950-954.

Sekiba K, Yoshida N, Awaji H, Fukaya T, Mitsuhashi N, Miyazaki K, Mizunuma H, Noda Y, Ono T, Osada H, Saji F, Sawada T, Sugimura K (1991): Multicenter study of interceed (TC7) absorbable adhesions barrier to reduce postoperative adhesion formation in infertility and endometriosis surgery. Obstet Gynecol (Tokyo) 58:1424-1432, and Int J Obstet Gynecol XIII World Congress of Gynaecology & Obstetrics (FIGO) Abstract #840.

Shimanuki T, Nishimura K, diZerega GS (1987): Localized prevention of postsurgical adhesion formation and reformation with oxidized regenerated cellulose. J Biomed Mat Res 21:173-185.

Soules MR, Dennis L, Bosarge A, Moore DE (1982): The prevention of postoperative pelvic adhesions: An animal study comparing barrier methods with dextran 70. Am J Obstet Gynecol 143:829-834.

Spagna PM, Peskin GW (1961): An experimental study of fibrinolysis in the prophylaxis of peritoneal adhesions. Surg Gynec Obstet 113:547-550.

Surrey MW, Friedman S (1982): Second-look laparoscopy after reconstructive pelvic surgery for infertility. J Reprod Med 27:658-660.

Swolin K (1966): Experimentelle Studien zur Prophylaxe von intraabdominalen Verwachsungen: Versuche an der Ratte mit einer Emulsion aus Lipid und Prednisolon. Acta Obstet Gynec Scand 45:473-498.

Thomas JW, Rhoads JE (1950): Adhesions resulting from removal of serosa from an area of bowel: failure of "oversewing" to lower incidence in the rat and the guinea pig. Arch Surg 61:565-576.

Thompson JN, Paterson-Brown S, Harbourne T, Whawell SA, Kalodiki E, Dudley HA (1989): Reduced human peritoneal plasminogen activating activity: possible mechanism of adhesion formation. Br J Surg 76:382-384.

Trimbos-Kemper TCM, Trimbos JB, van Hall EV (1985): Adhesion formation after tubal surgery: results of the eighth-day laparoscopy in 188 patients. Fertil Steril 43:395-400.

Trusler JK (1931): Peritonities: an experimental model of healing in the peritoneum and the therapeutic effort of amniotic fluid concentrate. Arch Surg 22:983-992.

Tulandi T (1990): Treatment-dependent and treatment-independent pregnancy among women with periadnexal adhesions. Am J Obstet Gynecol 162:354-357.

Turunen AOI (1933): Über die postoperativen Verwachs Ungen und deren Verhutung speziell im Anschluss an gynakologische Laparotomien. Duodecim Ser B 18:1-9.

Warren S (1928): The effects of amniotic fluid on serous surfaces. Arch Path 6:860-866.

Weibel M-A, Majno G (1973): Peritoneal adhesions and their relation to abdominal surgery. Am J Surg 126:345-353.

Wiseman DM, Gottlick LE, Diamond (1991): Haemostasis at a bleeding site using thrombin and the efficacy of Interceed absorbable adhesion barrier with and without heparin. International Society for Gynaecologic Endoscopy, Barcelona, Spain, October 1991. Abstract: Operative laporoscopy.

Yemini M, Meshorer A, Katz Z, Rozenman D, Lancet M (1984): Prevention of reformation of pelvic adhesions by "barrier" methods. Int J Fertil 29:194-196.

Zachariae L (1954): Hydrocortisone acetate applied intraperitoneally. I. Inhibitory effect on adhesions produced by telc. Acta Endocr 16:149-159.

Gynecologic Surgery and Adhesion Prevention, pages 19–44

ENDOMETRIOSIS, MACROPHAGES, AND ADHESIONS

A.F. Haney, M.D.
Division of Reproductive Endocrinology & Infertility
Department of Obstetrics and Gynecology
Duke University Medical Center
Durham, NC 27710

INTRODUCTION

Wound healing is a complex process involving not only the connective tissue and epithelial cells present at the site of injury but also platelets, fibroblasts and immune cells resident and elicited into the area. This is an orderly process which involves paracrine regulation by cytokines and growth factors, as well as hemostatic mechanisms which control deposition and lysis of fibrin. Each anatomic site has intrinsic characteristics which determine the pattern of the wound repair. Furthermore, variations in the local environment present at the time of injury may modify this response. The specific pattern of healing depends upon the nature of the injury, the number and level of activation of the immune cells present at that locale, the vascularity of the tissue and the presence of any previous or continuing pro-inflammatory stimuli.

The peritoneal cavity is unusual in that it contains a large resident population of immune cells with a wide range of biologic activities which have the potential to modify the pattern of tissue response to injury. Many of our concepts of wound healing are based on experimental paradigms of surgical injury, most frequently involving the skin. This is a very attractive model because of the uniformity of the tissue, the ease in evaluating experimental endpoints and the ability to precisely control the variables known to influence skin healing. Furthermore, a similar skin healing response across different species gives any result a high likelihood of clinical applicability because of the pressing concern of healing surgical incisions. Site-specific responses, however, must be considered when clinically evaluating tissue healing and any adjunctive treatments designed to modify the pattern of tissue repair.

ANATOMY OF THE PERITONEUM

The parietal and visceral peritoneum is composed of a single layer of surface cells, the so-called "mesothelial" cells, attached to a basement membrane which overlies a relatively avascular extracellular matrix and underlying smooth muscle (Hertzler, 1919; Pfeiffer, et al., 1987). The exact origin of the mesothelial cells is uncertain, but they resemble the cells lining the pleural cavity both functionally and morphologically.

Not only is the peritoneum physically very dissimilar from the skin, but the pattern of tissue repair is dramatically different. The length of time for healing a skin wound is proportional to the size of the injury, i.e., the distance between the edges of the wound. The peritoneum, regardless of the size of the injury, heals in the same time interval, 5 to 7 days (Ellis, et al., 1965; Hubbard, et al., 1967; Raftery, 1973a-c). These observations reinforce the concept that wound healing varies by the organ involved and that each site must be considered unique and evaluated separately. The postoperative scarring which concerns the gynecologic surgeon generally involves coalescing adhesions between the visceral and parietal peritoneum. This is a critical issue for women desirous of future reproduction as even miminal adnexal adhesions may reduce oocyte pick-up by the fallopian tubes.

THE PERITONEAL ENVIRONMENT

The Peritoneal Fluid

The peritoneal cavity normally contains a small volume of straw-colored fluid which serves a lubricating function for the mobile intraperitoneal viscera. In men, women after hysterectomy and women suppressing ovulation with oral steroids, there is typically 3 to 5 mL of peritoneal fluid {PF} (Mathuis, et al., 1978; Van Furth, et al., 1979). In normally menstruating women, there are somewhat larger PF volumes which vary during the menstrual cycle, being largest at the time of ovulation, often reaching 15 to 20 mL. (see review: Hurst and Rock, 1991)

The higher PF volume in normal cycling women likely can be attributed to the fact that the PF appears to be a combination of a transudate of serum and an exudate of the ovary with an uncertain contribution being secreted from the peritoneal lining itself. The exudate from the ovary is reflected in the extemely high levels of gonadal steroids in the PF, paralleling the dominant cyclic structure present on the ovary (Koninckx, et al., 1980). Some contribution may also come from regurgitated menses as bloody PF is virtually a universal event in cycling women with patent fallopian tubes (Blumenkrantz, et al., 1981; Halme, et al., 1984). The retrograde menstruation probably only occurs with ovulatory menses as the pressure within the uterus necessary to overcome that of the utero-tubal junction is created by prostaglandin-mediated uterine contractions with the prostanoids secreted by decidualized endometrium.

The Peritoneal Fluid Cell Population

The resident PF cell population is composed primarily of large mononuclear cells with all the morphologic and functional characteristics of tissue macrophages (Haney, et al., 1981; Halme, et al., 1982; Badaway, et al., 1984; Chacho, et al., 1986; Syrop and Halme, 1987; see review: Hurst and Rock, 1991). A smaller number of lymphocytes is present with most, if not all, subsets of lymphocytes represented (Hill, et al., 1988). Unless an acute infection is present, there are only rare polymorphonuclear leukocytes in the PF. Surprisingly, it is rare to identify true mesothelial cells on PF cytology, despite the frequent comment from cyto-pathologists regarding the presence of "reactive mesothelial cells" in the PF. While it has little clinical importance in screening for the presence of a malignancy, these cells are PF macrophages based on their morphology, positive staining for esterase and peroxidase (Haney, et al., 1981) and their phagocytic capability (Haney, et al., 1983).

In an analogous fashion to the PF volume, the PF leukocyte count is higher in normally cycling women than in men, women without a uterus and women suppressing ovarian function pharmacologically. These cells appear to play a role as part of a normal host defense system for the female genital tract, which, by the very nature of human reproduction, must come into contact with the environment, i.e., semen.

Rapid phagocytosis of human sperm _in vitro_ by PF macrophages collected from women has been reported (Muscato, et al., 1982). This may be helpful in removing sperm from the peritoneal cavity where fertilization and embryo development are not desirable events. Furthermore, semen is not sterile and all but a single spermatozoa will not be involved in actual fertilization. This is a well-designed peritoneal defense system activated by the onset of ovulatory cycles at puberty with the function of protecting women from the peritoneal contamination accompanying coitus and menstruation. These phagocytic cells may also function to remove other debris contaminating the female genital tract which migrates via the fallopian tubes into the abdomen.

ENDOMETRIOSIS AND ADHESIONS

Women with endometriosis have long been suspected of having an increased propensity for postoperative pelvic adhesions, albeit based on little other than anecdotal data. The findings of extensive peritoneal scarring around ectopic endometrial implants, frequent adhesions between a normal ovary and pelvic sidewall implants, compromise of the bowel lumen by the excessive fibrosis surrounding serosal implants and the occasional patient with ureteral obstruction secondary to retroperitoneal fibrosis (Haney, 1987) have tended to reinforce the clinical impression that women with endometriosis have a tendency toward exaggerated scarring.

The reason for any increase in peritoneal scarring in these women remains to be elucidated. A prime candidate would be the impact of a heightened degree of PF inflammation on the peritoneal healing response. The PF with its complement of immunologically active cells is in intimate and constant contact with the peritoneal surfaces directly interacting with the cells involved with tissue repair.

INTRAPERITONEAL INFLAMMATION IN WOMEN WITH ENDOMETRIOSIS

A sterile PF inflammatory process has long been observed in infertile women with endometriosis (see review: Hurst and Rock, 1991). This is manifested by higher PF volumes, protein concentrations and leukocyte numbers as well as an increase in the percentage of functionally activated macrophages. These cells secrete increased quantities of a diverse group of factors commonly found at the site of inflammation. These include prostanoids, proteolytic enzymes, lysozyme, cytokines and growth factors (Table 1). In addition, ectopic endometrium has the potential to elaborate a wide variety of cytokines as the endometrium is a site of active cytokine production (Tabibzadeh, 1991). The PF inflammatory process appears to be localized as there are no alterations in the pattern of circulating leukocytes (Gleicher, et al., 1984) nor alterations in the plasma levels of acute phase reactants synthesized by the liver (Dunselman, et al., 1988). Furthermore, there are no systemic clinical manifestations of this PF exudate and, aside from their infertility, these are asymptomatic women.

TABLE 1: SOLUBLE FACTORS KNOWN TO BE PRESENT IN THE PERITONEAL FLUID OF INFERTILE WOMEN WITH ENDOEMTRIOSIS

LYSOZYME	elevated in infertile women with no mechanical compromize of the pelvic pelvic viscera, including those with endometriosis
PROSTANOIDS ACID PHOSPHATASE NEUTRAL PROTEASE TUMOR NECROSIS FACTOR INTERLEUKIN-1 INTERLEUKIN-6	elevated in women with endometriosis
$ALPHA_2$-MACRO-GLOBULIN	altered bio:immuno ratio in women with endometriosis
PLATELET DERIVED GROWTH FACTOR FIBRONECTIN	increased secretion by PF macrophages, *in vitro* from women with endometriosis
MONOCYTE/MACRO-PHAGE COLONY STIMULATING FACTOR	elevated in women with several types of gynecologic pathology including endometriosis

The only intrinsic immune alteration postulated in women with endometriosis is that of a unique cell-mediated immune deficiency directed toward endometrial cells. This is based upon two observations, a reduced number of leukocytes infiltrating around experimentally-implanted subcutaneous endometrium in monkeys with spontaneous pelvic endometriosis (Dmowski, et al., 1981) and an endometriosis-dependent suppression of lymphocyte-mediated lysis of autologous endometrial cells, _in vitro_ (Steele, et al., 1984). It has recently been suggested that the lymphocytes involved in this phenomenon are natural killer cells (Oosterlynck, et al., 1991). However, no immune deficiencies have been observed in women with endometriosis as would have been anticipated in the presence of depressed natural killer cell activity.

The Stimulus Responsible

Initially, it was thought that the inflammatory stimulus responsible for eliciting this exudate was debris from cycling ectopic endometrium. Most visible implants, however, are completely encapsulated by collagen and effectively retroperitonealized (Haney, 1987). As a consequence, the implants are not in continuity with the PF and the menstrual debris is entrapped, giving the implants their typical blue-grey appearance, the so-called "powderburn". There is little evidence that ectopic endometrium is able to respond to gonadal steroids in a fashion comparable to intrauterine endometrium (Metzger, et al., 1988). Similarly, the luteal phase endometrial secretory product, prolactin, is not increased in the PF of women with endometriosis (Haney, et al., 1984). These observations suggest that peritoneal endometrial implants have only a limited potential to contribute soluble factors and menstrual debris to the PF.

Virtually all women retrograde menstruate every cycle (Blumenkrantz, et al., 1981; Halme, et al., 1984) and viable endometrial cells can be cultured from the PF in most women with the greatest number of viable cells noted immediately following menses

(Kruitwagen, et al., 1991). Interestingly, there is not a greater number of endometrial cells identified in the PF of women with endometriosis. This is consistent with the finding that PF inflammation is present in virtually all infertile women without a mechanical cause for their infertility (Olive, et al., 1987). When menstrual cycles are suppressed, the parameters of PF inflammation are dramatically reduced (Haney and Weinberg, 1988). Furthermore, the magnitude of the PF inflammation, as judged by the PF volume and leukocyte count, is inversely correlated with the amount of endometriosis (Haney, et al., 1991). Hence, the identification of ectopic endometrium in the peritoneal cavity appears to be a coincidental finding in these women, and the real culprit is retrograde menstruation and the peritoneal cavity's immunological response.

There are two possible explanations for the impressive PF exudate in this sub-group of infertile women. First, these women may have a greater volume of regurgitated menstrual debris and a proportionally larger peritoneal inflammatory reaction. Unfortunately, there is no technique available to quantify the amount of menstrual effluent regurgitated into the peritoneal cavity. The second possibility is that these women could have an exaggerated PF immune response to "normal" retrograde menstruation. A unique PF immune response could be attributable to some unidentified factor within the menstrual debris or a genetic predisposition. At present, these possibilities cannot be separated.

PERITONEAL FLUID INFLAMMATION AND WOUND HEALING

Women with a PF inflammatory exudate have the potential for an altered pattern of postoperative wound healing as a result of the impact of the exudate on the cells involved in wound repair. This would be roughly analogous to performing a surgical procedure at the site of an ongoing pro-inflammatory stimulus such as a foreign body reaction or a soft tissue infection except that the inflammation is in the PF which is in intimate contact with any peritoneal injuries. In these circumstances, there will be a large number of activated leukocytes present at that site with increased levels of a wide variety of soluble products secreted by these cells (Bryant, et al., 1988). These factors act as autocrine and paracrine regulators of the tissue repair.

Paradoxically, the elicitation of macrophages at a post-inflammatory peritoneal repair site may serve a helpful function as well. An increase in the PF leukocytes is part of the normal postsurgical repair process. It has been observed in children with peritonitis that those with a normal macrophage component to their peritoneal exudate have fewer postoperative adhesions (Kharin, 1990). In this circumstance, the normal function of mononuclear phagocytes is likely required for the removal of cellular debris to allow peritoneal healing to occur without adhesions. The relationship between immune cells and wound repair cells is undoubtedly a complex one and each clinical situation must be viewed as unique. The tissue response to a surgical injury, for instance, may have a different outcome if it is the cause of the entrance of macrophages into the peritoneal cavity as contrasted to the healing response when surgery is performed in the midst of an ongoing inflammatory process. In both circumstances, increased numbers of PF macrophages will be present during healing, but the tissue repair may be dramatically different.

Immunomodulatory Cytokines

Interleukin-1 The interaction of pro-inflammatory cytokines with tissue repair cells has the potential to alter the healing response. Interleukin-1 (IL-1) is known to be elevated in the PF of women with endometriosis (Fakih, et al., 1987) and IL-1 stimulates fibroblast proliferation, collagen deposition and fibrinogen formation (Schmidt, et al, 1982; Postlewaite, et al., 1984; Freundlich, et al., 1986). In a rodent model of adhesion formation, intraperitoneal injection of IL-1 increased the number and severity of adhesion formation (Hershlag, et al., 1991). Additionally, IL-1 treatment of endothelial cells decreases the production of tissue fibrinolytic activity and increases the production of cell-associated procoagulant activity as well as a specific inhibitor to fibrinolytic activity (Bevilacqua, et al., 1986). These IL-1 stimulated events would be expected to enhance the deposition of collagen and increase the potential for significant scarring. This has led to the suggestion that the elevated PF IL-1 is responsible for the adhesions and peritoneal fibrosis in women with endometriosis.

<u>Interleukin-6</u> Interleukin-6 (IL-6) is a potent cytokine having diverse effects, several of which are potentially related to tissue repair, including stimulation of acute phase reactant synthesis by hepatocytes (Gauldie, et al., 1987), angiogenesis (Motro, et al., 1990) and paracrine/auatocrine stimulation of tumor cells (Kirnbauer, et al., 1989), including ovarian cancer cells (Watson, et al., 1990). Furthermore, IL-6 is secreted by monocytes/macrophages (Gauldie, et al., 1987) and has been noted to be elevated in women with endometriosis (Buyalos, et al., 1991). Additional work will be necessary in order to evaluate a possible impact of IL-6 on the pathophysiology of endometriosis and wound healing.

<u>Tumor Necrosis Factor</u> Tumor necrosis factor (TNF), another cytokine with a wide range of biologic effect, is known to be elevated in the PF of women with endometriosis (Eisermann, et al., 1988). Human peritoneal macrophages have been noted to secrete TNF, <u>in vitro</u>, with those collected from women with endometriosis having the greatest production rate (Halme, 1989). The two forms of TNF, TNF-alpha or cachexin and TNF-beta or lyphotoxin, are both inflammatory mediators exhibiting cytotoxic activity against tumor cells, stimulating production of growth factors such as hematopoietic growth factor and, importantly, inducing fibroblast proliferation (Broudy, et al.,

1987). These are both very potent cytokines and the presence of increased levels of TNF in the PF of women with endometriosis suggests it may explain an altered tissue response to injury or endometriosis-associated scarring.

Plasminogen Activator Plasminogen activator (PA) is a trypsin-like proteinase found in high concentrations in many extracellular fluids which causes cleavage of plasminogen to plasmin leading to the breakdown of fibrin. Cultured monocytes and macrophages (Saksela, et al., 1985) and activated peritoneal macrophages (Orita, et al., 1986) secrete PA as well as protease inhibitors (Fukasawa, et al., 1989) which inactivate urokinase-like PA activity. This balance between clotting and clot lysis is extremely important in wound repair as the prolonged presence of a fibrin matrix at the site of injury acts as a framework for fibroblasts to infiltrate the site and lay down collagen. The net result is that the fibrin acts like a "glue" between injured peritoneal surfaces and increases the likelihood of forming permanent coalescing adhesions (Buckman, et al., 1976). The prompt lysis of the fibrin matrix, by plasmin, is essential to reduce this adhesiogenic stimulus. In experimental animal models, the use of recombinant tissue plasminogen activator reduces the development of peritoneal adhesions (Doody, et al., 1989; Dorr, et al, 1990). Whether this approach will prove beneficial clinically is unclear at present, but further animal data should be forthcoming.

A 50% or greater reduction in plasminogen activator activity can prevent the elimination of fibrin, and such a reduction in plasminogen activity has been suggested to be the cause of adhesions in women with endometriosis (Malick, 1982). However, plasminogen activator activity in the PF has not been found to be lower in women with endometriosis nor is there a correlation with the stage of the disease (Batzofin, et al., 1985). Clinical trials with tissue plasminogen activator will be necessary to confirm this hypothesis, if only as an adjunct for the prevention of postoperative adhesions.

Alpha$_2$-Macroglobulin Alpha$_2$-macroglobulin, a large proteinase inhibitor secreted by macrophages, has been found in the PF of women (Hoffman, et al., 1988; Dunselman, et al., 1988). While the PF levels of immunoreactive alpha$_2$-macroglobulin are not altered in the presence of endometriosis, a reduction in biologic activity was noted (Hoffman, et al, 1988). What effect the change in the bio:immuno ratio of this major proteinase inhibitor will have on the activity of the various proteinase substrates in PF, specifically PA, remains to be determined. It is not clear whether this change is specific for endometriosis or whether this is typical of PF in the presence of a PF exudate.

Trypsin Inhibitor Activity Women with endometriosis have been noted to have increased trypsin inhibitory activity in their PF during the luteal phase (Fazleabas, et al., 1987). The two major proteinase inhibitors expected to be present in the PF are alpha$_1$-antitrypsin and alpha$_2$-macroglobulin and these are also acute phase reactants. The contributions of each of these proteinase inhibitors to the total trypsin inhibitor activity in PF is not known but other investigators have noted no difference in the levels of alpha$_2$-macroglobulin (Hoffman, et al., 1988; Dunselman, et al., 1988) or alpha$_1$-antitrypsin (Dunselman, et al., 1988) in the PF of women with endometriosis. There was a discrepancy noted in the amount biologically active and immunologically detectable alpha$_2$-macroglobulin in the PF of women with endometriosis (Hoffman, et al., 1988), further confusing the issue as to what was responsible for the increase in trypsin inhibitor activity. Possible explanations may be the fact that the two studies which did not note an increase did not separate the follicular and luteal values and that the PF exudate is comparable in women with minimal endometriosis and "idiopathic" infertility. Clarifcation of these issues will require careful study of PF parameters considering the stage of the cycle, the presence of PF inflammation independent of visible endometiosis and the possiblitiy of other unidentified proteinase inhibitors.

Growth Factors

Several of the so-called growth factors have been indentified in the PF of women both with and without endometiosis. This group of paracrine and autocrine hormones is important in wound healing as they serve to not only stimulate the proliferation and function of the classic tissue repair cell, the fibroblast, but also to induce angiogenesis in the wound (Takemura and Werb, 1984; Bryant, et al., 1988). Furthermore, growth factors have been suggested to be involved in the pathogenesis of endometriosis itself by increasing the likelihood that free-floating endometrial cells will survive and attach to the peritoneal surface (Halme, et al, 1987).

Platelet-Derived Growth Factor A growth factor was previously identified in the PF of women with endometriosis, based on a bioassay (Halme, et al, 1988a). This was originally thought unique to the peritoneal cavity and was termed "macrophage-derived growth factor". Subsequently, this molecule was found to be identical to platelet-derived growth factor (PDGF). PDGF is secreted by PF macrophages in vitro with increasing secretory activity positively correlated with the stage of the disease (Halme, 1988b). On the basis of the increased PDGF secretion by activated macrophages, it was suggested that the regurgitated endometrial cells have a greater probability of survival and adherence on the peritoneal surface. It would be reasonable to consider a similar mechanism might be operative with tissue repair cells in the peritoneum. In support of this concept, human mesothelial cells have been shown to undergo mitosis in response to PDGF, in vitro (Gabrielson, et al., 1988), which is unusual for epithelial cells but typical for connective tissue cells. The presence of this paracrine factor in the PF in intimate contact with tissue repair cells in a peritoneal defect may have a similar effect.

Epidermal Growth Factor The protein hormone epidermal growth factor (EGF) is widely distributed in the body and has now been identified in the PF of women (DeLeon, et al., 1986). EGF levels in the PF are positively correlated with the day of the cycle with overall higher levels in the luteal phase compared to the follicular phase. The concentrations were not, however, different in women with endometriosis and did not correlate with prostaglandin levels, despite the fact that EGF is known to release prostanoids in other tissues.

EGF acts as a mitogen for most epithelial cells and EGF receptors have a wide distribution, including mesenchymal cells. Importantly, in a wound healing context, EGF has now been demonstrated to synergize with PDGF to cause proliferation of fibroblasts. Whether EGF has an impact on the development or pattern of scarring with endometriosis is unclear but EGF is both synthesized and acts in the endometrium and presumably endometrial implants. Until more data are available, this will simply be considered as a growth factor present in PF with the potential to alter the tissue response to injury.

Macrophage Colony Stimulating Factor Another growth factor, macrophage colony stimulating factor (M-CSF), has been identified in the PF of women at consistently higher concentrations than in plasma (Weinberg, et al., 1991). The total PF M-CSF is higher in women with endometriosis but also in women with other types of gynecologic pathology compared to fertile women and, hence, appears to be a non-specific indicator of gynecologic pathology. While the M-CSF could be secreted by fibroblasts, mesothelial cells or endothelial cells, the levels of M-CSF are positively correlated with the number of PF macrophages suggesting they are the source of the M-CSF in PF. Interestingly, M-CSF is also secreted by endometrial cells (Azuma, et al., 1990) and either endometriosis or the free-floating endometrial cells in the PF may be another source of M-CSF. This growth factor is involved in both the differentiation of monocytes to become phenotypically "activated" macrophages and it can serve as a chemotatic factor for blood monocytes. M-CSF may play a role in eliciting the leukocytes into the peritoneal cavity as well as altering their activity. It has the potential to exert auto-regulatory control on the PF cell population which may be altered in pathologic situations.

<u>Fibronectin</u> One of the components of extracellular matrix, fibronectin is a high molecular weight glycoprotein present in a free form plasma and other body fluids. It is secreted by a number of cell types, including pulmonary alveolar macrophages, and has a wide range of biologic activities including that of a growth factor for fibroblasts, an immunomodulator of macrophages and a cell adhesion molecule important in cell migration. Fibronectin has been identified in the PF of women with endometriosis but the concentrations are lower than in women without the disease (Kauma, et al., 1988). This molecule is secreted by PF macrophages, <u>in vitro</u>, and in substantially greater quantities when endometriosis is present. Whether this has any role to play in either the pathophysiology of endometriosis or peritoneal scarring remains speculative, but it should be considered in these contexts.

<u>Fibroblast/Endometrial Stromal Cell Stimulating Factors</u> Macrophage-conditioned media has long been known to stimulate the proliferation and growth of fibroblasts (Leibovich and Ross, 1976; Bitterman, et al., 1982; Leslie, et al., 1984; Fukasawa, et al., 1987). PF from patients with endometriosis stimulates proliferation of endometrial stromal cells to a greater extent than PF from women without endometriosis (Surrey and Halme, 1990). An uncharacterized macrophage-derived growth factor has recently been described in an animal model which functions as a competence factor, allowing endometrial stromal cells to respond to mitogenic stimuli (Olive, et al., 1991). If a similar growth

factor is secreted by human macrophages, this may facilitate the growth of the stromal component of endometrial implants and the surrounding fibroproliferative response. Angiogenesis is also stimulated by factor(s) secreted by macrophages (Wissler, et al., 1986).

Interestingly, it has recently been observed that human PF contains a protein which induces the proliferation of endometrial-like cells _in vitro_ in a dose-response fashion in the absence of serum (Koutsilieris, et al., 1991). This factor stimulated fibroblasts and endometrial adenocarcinoma cells as well but had the greatest effect on rabbit endometrial cells. This activity was identical in the PF from women with and without endometriosis so it appears to be a normal constituient of PF. Whether this activity is derived from PF macrophages was not investigated, but the material did have chemical differences from previously described growth factor found in the endometrium (Koutsilieris, 1990). It is not known if this factor will have an effect on wound healing, but it has the potential to increase the likelihood of establishing endometrial implants.

EFFECT OF IMMUNOMODULATION ON ADHESION FORMATION

It will be difficult to evaluate the impact of immunologically active cells on wound healing in the peritoneal cavity. One method to establish a relationship is to attempt to reduce the rate of adhesion formation by altering leukocyte number or function. While there are no data available in humans, several intriguing studies in animals suggest this may be a worthwhile avenue of research.

The first experiments involved depleting experimental animals of macrophages and it was noted their skin wounds had delayed healing (Leibovich and Ross, 1975). Subsequently, the immunomodulator pentoxyfilline (Steinleitner et al., 1989a) and an indigenous agent with immunostimulant properties, _asparagus racemosus_

(Rege, et al., 1989), were observed to reduce postoperative abdominal adhesions in separate experimental animal models. Additional studies using calcium channel blockade, which may act via its effects on immune cells, demonstrated a reduction in postsurgical adhesion formation in an animal paradigm (Steinleitner, et al., 1988; Steinleitner, et al., 1989b). One of the most significant secretory products of activated macrophages are superoxide anions which are largely responsible for their tumoricidal activity and are increased in tissue repair cells (Fukasawa, et al., 1988). Treatment with trimetazidine, a scavenger of oxygen radicals, has been shown to reduce peritoneal adhesions in a rat model (Tsimoyiannis, et al., 1990). By contrast, the non-steroidal anti-inflammatory agent, ibuprofen (Holtz, 1982), the potent steroid dexamethasone combined with the anti-histamine promethazine (Replogle, et al., 1966), and the intraperitoneal instillation of 32% dextran 70, which inhibits lymphocyte and macrophage function (Rein and Hill, 1989), have all failed to consistently reduce adhesion formation. While these data are seemingly contradictory, problems with the uniqueness of each of the model systems as well as the pharmacokinetics of the agents make these experiments not directly comparable.

While the concept of using pharmacologic immunomodulation to control wound repair is tantilizing, the involvement of the immune system in wound repair is complex with immune cells playing different roles under varying conditions. The use of agents which simply alter the function of specific immune cells, such as macrophages or lymphocytes, is unlikely to be rewarding unless critical steps in the wound healing process can be targeted and effectively blocked without undue risk to appropriate surgical healing and other necessary immune functions. As the tissue repair in the peritoneal cavity is rapid and has unique features such as the contact with PF, it is potentially possible to alter the fibroproliferative response within the peritoneum without significantly altering incisional healing. In order for immunomodulators to be of clinical value, it will be necessary to identify agents or localized delivery systems which can modify the impact of PF inflammatory cells on peritoneal repair at doses which will not cause unwanted and potentially serious systemic complications.

SUMMARY

In the judgement of most experienced clinicians, women with endometriosis are particularly prone to postoperative adhesion formation. Coincidently, a localized sterile PF inflammatory process is present in these women, although not exclusively confined to those with visible endometrial implants. This PF exudate contains numerous growth factors and cytokines, most secreted by the large population of activated macrophages, which have the potential to alter the tissue repair response. To further evaluate this possibility, attention will need to be focused on the nature of the PF immune system, changes in the PF immune response in various gynecologic disease states and the impact of surgery.

REFERENCES

Azuma C, Saji F, Kimura T, Tokugwa Y, Takemura M, Samejima Y, Tanizawa O (1990): Steroid hormones induce macrophage colony-stimulating factor (MCSF) and MCSF receptor mRNAs in the human endometrium. J Mol Endocrinol 5:103-108.

Badaway SZA, Cuenca V, Marshall L, Munchback R, Rinas AC, Coble DA (1984): Cellular components in peritoneal fluid in infertile patients with and without endometriosis. Fertil Steril 42:704-708.

Batzofin JH, Holmes SD, Gibbons WE, Buttram VC Jr (1985): Peritoneal fluid plasminogen activator activity in endometriosis and pelvic adhesive disease. Fertil Steril 44:277-279.

Bevilacqua MP, Schleef RR, Gimbrone MA, Loskutoff DJ (1986): Regulation of fibrinolytic system of cultured human vascular endothelium by Interleukin 1. J Clin Invest 78:587-591.

Bitterman PB, Rennard SI, Hunninghake GW, Crystal RG (1982): Human alveolar macrophage growth factor for fibroblasts. J Clin Inves 70:806-822.

Blumenkrantz MJ, Gallager N, Bashore RA, Tenckhoff H (1981): Retrograde menstruation in women undergoing chronic peritoneal dialysis. Obstet Gynecol 57:677-670.

Broudy VC, Harlan JM, Adamson JW (1987): Disparate effects of tumor necrosis factor-alpha/cachectin and tumor necrosis factor-beta/lymphotoxin on hematopoietic growth factor production and neutrophil adhesion molecule expression by cultured human endothelial cells. J Immunol 138:4298-4302.

Bryant SM, Fukasawa M, Orita H, Rodgers KE, diZerega GS (1988): Mediation of post-surgical wound healing by macrophages. In "Growth Factors and Other Aspects of Wound Healing: Biological and Clinical Implications". Alan R. Liss, Inc., pp 273-290.

Buckman RF, Woods M, Sargent L, Gervin AS (1976): A unifying pathogenetic mechanism in the etiology of intraperitoneal adhesions. J Surg Res 20:1-5.

Buyalos RP, Funari VA, Azziz R, et al (1991): Elevated interleukin-6 levels in peritoneal fluid of patients with pelvic pathology. Abstract # 120, p. 158, presented at the 38th Annual meeting of the Society for Gynecologic Investigation, San Antonio, TX.

Chacho KJ, Stronkowski-Chacho M, Andressen PJ, Scommegna A (1986): Peritoneal fluid in patients with and without endometriosis: Prostanoids and macrophages and their effect on the spermatozoa penetration assay. Am J Obstet Gynecol 154:1290-1299.

DeLeon FD, Vijayakurnay R, Brown M, Rao ChV, Yussman MA, Schultz G (1986): Peritoneal fluid volume, estrogen, progesterone, prostaglandin, and epidermal growth factor concentrations in patients with and without endometriosis. Obstet Gynecol 68:189-194.

Dmowski WP, Steele RW, Baker GF (1981) : Deficient cellular immunity in endometriosis. Am J Obstet Gynecol 141:377-383.
Doody KJ, Dunn RC, Buttram VC Jr (1989): Recombinant tissue plasminogen activator reduces adhesion formation in a rabbit uterine horn model. Fertil Steril 51:509-512.
Dorr PJ, Vemer HN, Brommer EJ, Willemsen WN, Veldhuizen RW (1990): Prevention of postoperative adhesions by tissue-type plasminogen activator (t-PA) in the rabbit. European J Obstet Gynecol 37:287-291.
Dunselman GAJ, Bouckaert PXJM, Evers JLH (1988): The acute-phase response in endometriosis of women. J Reprod Fertil 83:803-808.
Eisermann J, Gast MJ, Pineda J, Odem RR, Collins JL (1988): Tumor necrosis factor in peritoneal fluid of women undergoing laparoscopic surgery. Fertil Steril 50:573-579.
Fakih H, Baggett B, Holtz G, Tsang KY, Lee JC, Williamson HO (1987): Interleukin-1: A possible role in the infertility associated with endometriosis. Fertil Steril 47:212-217.
Fazbeabas AT, Khan-Dawood FS, Dawood MY (1987): Proteins, progesterone, and protease inhibitors in uterine and peritoneal fluids of women with endometriosis. Fertil Steril 47:218-224.
Freundlich B, Bomalaski JS, Neilson E, Jimenez SA (1986): Regulation of fibroblast proliferation and collagen synthesis by cytokines. Immunol Today 7:303-307.
Fukasawa M, Bryant SM, Nakamura RM, diZerega GS (1987): Modulation of fibroblast proliferation by postsurgical macrophages. J Surg Res 43:513-520.
Fukasawa M, Bryant SM, diZerega GS (1988): Superoxide anion production by postsurgical macrophages. J Surg Res 45:382-388.
Fukasawa M, Bryant SM, Orita H, Campeau JD, diZerega GS (1989): Modulation of proline and glucosamine incorporation into tissue repair cells by peritoneal macrophages. J Surg Res 46:166-171.
Gabrielson EW, Gerwin BI, Harris CC, Roberts AB, Sporn MB (1988): Stimulation of DNA synthesis in

cultured primary human mesothelial cells by specific growth factors. Faseb J 2:2717- 2721.
Gauldie J, Richards C, Harnish D, Lansforp P, Baumann H (1987): Interferon b2/B cell stimulatory factor type 2 shares identity with monocyte-derived hepatocyte stimulating factor and regulates the major acute phase protein response in liver cells. Proc Nat Acad Sci USA 84:7251-7255.
Gleicher N, Dmowski WP, Seigel I, Liu TL, Friberg J, Radwanska E, Toder V (1984): Lymphocyte subsets in endometriosis. Obstet Gynecol 63:463-466.
Halme J, Becker S, Hammond MG, Raj S (1982): Pelvic macrophages in normal and infertile women: the role of patent tubes. Am J Obstet Gynecol 142:890-895.
Halme J, Hammond MG, Hulka JF (1984): Retrograde menstruation in healthy women and in patients with endometriosis. Obstet Gynecol 64:151-154.
Halme J, Becker S, Haskill S (1987): Altered maturation and function of peritoneal macrophages - possible role in pathogenesis of endometriosis. Am J Obstet Gynecol 156:783-789.
Halme J, White C, Kauma S, Haskill S (1988a): Peritoneal macrophages from patients with endometriosis release growth factor activity _in vitro_. J Clin Endocrinol Metab 66:1044-1049.
Halme J (1988b): Endometriosis-related peripheral macrophages release platelet derived growth factor in vitro. Fertil Steril 50:s33.
Halme J (1989): Release of tumor necrosis factor-alpha by human peritoneal macrophages in vivo and in vitro. Am J Obstet Gynecol 161:1718-1725.
Haney AF, Muscato JJ, Weinberg JB (1981): Peritoneal fluid cell populations in infertility patients. Fertil Steril 35:696-698.
Haney AF, Misukonis MA, Weinberg JB (1983): Macrophages and infertility: Oviductal macrophages as potential mediators of infertility. Fertil Steril 39:310-315.
Haney AF, Handwerger S, Weinberg JB (1984): Peritoneal fluid prolactin in infertile women with endometriosis: Lack of evidence of secretory

activity by endometrial implants. Fertil Steril 42:935-938.

Haney AF (1987): Pelvic endometriosis: Etiology and pathology. In Gondos B, Riddick DH (eds): "The Pathology of Infertility, New York: Theime-Stratton Inc., pp 85-100.

Haney AF, Weinberg JB (1988): Reduction of the intraperitoneal inflammation associated with endometriosis by treatment with medroxy-progesterone acetate. Am J Obstet Gynecol 159: 450-454.

Haney AF, Jenkins SJ, Weinberg JB (1991): The stimulus responsible for the peritoneal fluid inflammation observed in infertile women with endometriosis. Fertil Steril 56:408-413.

Hershlag A, Otterness IC, Bliven ML, Diamond MP, Polan ML (1991): The effect of interleukin-1 on adhesion formation in the rat. Am J Obstet Gynecol 165:771-774.

Hertzler AF (1919): "The Peritoneum." St. Louis: CV Mosby.

Hill JA, Faris HMP, Schiff I, Anderson DJ (1988): Characterization of leukocyte subpopulations in the peritoneal fluid of women with endometriosis. Fertil Steril 50:216-222.

Hoffman M, Haney AF, Weinberg JB (1988): Reduced trypsin-binding capacity of alpha2-macroglobulin in the peritoneal fluid of women with endometriosis: Possible relevence to alterations in macrophage function. Fertil Steril 50:39-47.

Holtz G, Baker E, Tsai C (1980): Effect of thirty-two percent dextran-70 on peritoneal adhesion formation and re-formation after lysis. Fertil Steril 33:660-662.

Holtz G (1982): Failure of a nonsteroidal anti-inflammatory agent (ibuprofen) to inhibit peritoneal adhesion reformation after lysis. Fertil Steril 37:582-583.

Hurst BS, Rock JA (1991): The peritoneal environment in endometriosis. In Thomas EJ, Rock JA (eds): "Modern Approaches to Endometriosis." Boston: Kluwer Academic Publishers, pp 79-96.

Kauma S, Clark MR, White C, Halme J (1988): Production of fibronectin by peritoneal macrophages and concentrations of fibronectin in peritoneal fluid from patients with and without endometriosis. Obstet Gynecol 72:13-18.

Kharin G (1990): The role of the mononuclear phagocyte system in the pathogenesis of excessive peritoneal adhesions in children with peritonitis. Pediatriia 8:49-51.

Kirnbauer R, Kock A, Schwartz T, Urbanski A, Krutmann J, Borth W, Damm D, Shipley G, Ansel JC, Luger TA (1989): INF-b2, B cell differentiation factor 3, or hybirdoma growth factor (LI-6) is expressed and released by human epidermal cells and epidermoid carcinoma cell lines. J Immunol 142:1922-1928.

Koninckx PR, Raner M, Brosens IA (1980): Origin of peritoneal fluid in women: an ovarian exudation product. Br J Obstet Gynaecol 87:177-183.

Koutsilieris M (1990): Uterus-derived growth substances: Possible implications for human uterus physiology and pathophysiology (Review). In Vitro 4:45-48.

Koutsilieris M, Allaire-Michaud L, Fortier M, Lemay A (1991): Mitogen(s) for endometrial-like cells can be detected in human peritoneal fluid. Fertil Steril 56:888-893.

Kruitwagen RFMP, Poels LG, Willemsen WNP, de Ronde IJY, Jap PHK, Rolland R (1991): Endometrial epithelial cells in peritoneal fluid during the early follicular phase. Fertil Steril 55:297-303.

Leibovich SJ, Ross R (1975): The role of macrophage in wound repair. A study with hydrocortisone and anti-macrophage serum. Am J Pathol 78:71-100.

Leibovich SJ, Ross R (1976): A macrophage-dependent factor that stimulates the proliferation of fibroblasts in vitro. Am J Pathol 84:501-514.

Leslie CC, Musson RS, Henson PM (1984): Production of growth factor activity for fibroblasts by human monocyte-derived macrophages. J Leukoc Biol 36:143-159.

Malick JE (1982): The etiology of endometriosis. J Am Osteopath Assoc 81:407-412.

Mathuis JB, Van Look PFA, Michie EA (1978): Changes in volume, total protein and ovarian steroid concentrations of peritoneal fluid throughout the human menstrual cycle. J Endocrinol 76:123-133.

Metzger DA, Olive DL, Haney AF (1988): Altered hormonal responsiveness of ectopic endometrium: Histologic correlation with intrauterine endometrium. Human Path 19:1417-1424.

Motro B, Itin A, Sachs L, Keshet E (1990): Pattern of interleukin-6 gene expression in vivo suggests a role for this cytokine in angiogenesis. Proc Nat Acad Sci USA 87:3092-3096.

Muscato JJ, Haney AF, Weinberg JB (1982): Sperm phagocytosis by human peritoneal macrophages: A possible cause of infertility in endometriosis. Am J Obstet Gynecol 144:503-510.

Olive DL, Haney AF, Weinberg JB (1987): The nature of the intraperitoneal exudate associated with infertility: Peritoneal fluid and serum lysozyme activity. Fertil Steril 48:802-806.

Olive DL, Montoya I, Riehl RM, Schenken RS (1991): Macrophage-conditioned media enhance endometrial stromal cell proliferation in vitro. Am J Obstet Gynecol 164:953-958.

Oosterlynck DJ, Cornillie FJ, Waer M, Vandeputte M, Koninckx PR (1991): Women with endometriosis show a defect in natural killer cell activity resulting in decreased cytotoxicity to autologous endometrium. Fertil Steril 56:45-51.

Orita H, Campeau, Gale JA, Nakamura RM, diZerega GS (1986): Differential secretion of plasminogen activator activity by postsurgical activated macrophages. J Surg Res 41:569-573.

Pfeiffer CJ, Pfeiffer DC, Misra HP (1987): Enteric serosal surface in the piglet. A scanning and transmission electron microscopic study of the mesothelium. J Submicrosc Cytol 19:237-246.

Postlewaite AE, Lachman LB, Kang AH (1984): Induction of fibroblast proliferation by interleukin-1 derived from human monocytic leukemic cells. Arthritis Rheum 27:995-1001.

Raftery AT (1973a). Regeneration of parietal and visceral peritoneum: An electron microscopical study. J Anat 115:375-392.

Raftery AT (1973b). Regeneration of parietal and visceral peritoneum: A light microscopical study. Br J Surg 60:293-299.

Raftery AT: (1973c). Regeneration of parietal and visceral peritoneum in the immature animal: A light and electron microscopical study. Br J Surg 60:969-975.

Rege NN, Nazareth HM, Isaac A, Karandikar SM, Dahanukar SA (1989): Immunotherapeutic modulation of intraperitoneal adhesions by Asparagus racemosus. J Postgrad Med 35:199-203.

Rein MS, Hill JA (1989): 32% dextran 70 (Hyskon) inhibits lymphocyte and macrophage function in vitro: a potential new mechanism for adhesion prevention. Fertil Steril 52:953-957.

Replogle RL, Johnson R, Gross RE (1966): Prevention of postoperative intestinal adhesions with combined prometazine and dexamethasone therapy: Experimental and clinical studies. Ann Surg 163:580-588.

Saksela O, Houi T, Vaheri A (1985): Urokinase-type plasminogen activator and its inhibitor secreted by cultured human monocyte-macrophages. J Cell Physiol 122:125-132.

Schmidt JA, Mizel SB, Cohen D, GReen I (1982): Interleukin I, a potential regulator of fibroblast proliferation. J Immunol 128:2177-2182.

Steele RW, Dmowski WP, Marmer DJ (1984): Immunologic aspects of human endometriosis. Am J Reprod Immunol 6:33-36.

Steinleitner A, Lambert H, Montoro L, Kelly E, Swanson J, Sueldo C (1988): The use of calcium channel blockade for the prevention of postoperative adhesion formation. Fertil Steril 50:818-821.

Steinleitner A, Lambert H, Kazensky C, Danks P, Roy S (1989a): Use of pentoxyfylline as an adjuvant to prevent postsurgical adhesion formation: Preliminary investigations in a rodent model. J Gynecol Surg 5:367-373.

Steinleitner A, Kazensky C, Lambert H (1989b): Calcium channel blockade prevents postsurgical reformation of adnexal adhesions in rabbits. Obstet Gynecol 74:796-798.

Surrey ES, Halme J (1990): Effect of peritoneal fluid from endometriosis patients on endometrial stromal cell proliferation in vitro. Obstet Gynecol 76:792-797.

Syrop CH, Halme J (1987): Cyclic changes of peritoneal fluid parameters in normal and infertile patients. Obstet Gynecol 69:416-418.

Tabibzadeh S (1991): Human endometrium: An active site of cytokine production and action. Endocrin Rev 12:272-290.

Takemura R, Werb Z (1984): Secretory products of macrophages and their physiological functions. Am J Physiol 246:c1-9.

Tsimoyiannis EC, Lekkas ET, Paizis JB, Boulis SA, Page P, Kotoulas OB (1990): Prevention of peritoneal adhesions in rats with trimetazidine. Acta Chirurgica Scandinavica 156:771-774.

Van Furth R, Raeburn JA, Van Zwet TL (1979): Characteristics of human mononuclear phagocytes. Blood 54:485-500.

Watson JM, Sensintaffor JL, Bereck JS, Martinez-Maza O (1990): Constituitive production of IL-6 by ovarian cancer cell lines and by primary ovarian tumor cultures. Cancer Res 50:6959-6965.

Weinberg JB, Haney AF, Xu FJ, Ramakrishnan S (1991): Peritoneal fluid and plasma levels of human macrophage colony-stimulating factor in relation to peritoneal fluid macrophage content. Blood 78:513-516.

Wissler JH, Logemann E, Meyer HE, Krutzfeld B, Hockel M, Heilmeyer LMG (1986): Structure and function of a monocytic blood vessel morphogen (angiotropin) for angiogenesis in vivo and in vitro: A copper-containing metallo-polyribo-nucleo-polypeptide as a movel and unique type of monokine. Protides Biol Fluids 34:525-536.

Gynecologic Surgery and Adhesion Prevention, pages 45–49

ELECTROMICROSURGERY

Kurt Swolin
Department of Obstetrics and Gynecology
Sahlgrenska Hospital
The University of Göteborg
S-413 45 Göteborg, Sweden

With regard to electromicrosurgery, one can pose the questions why, when and how.

Firstly, why? The reason for development of the technique was to improve the results obtained with infertility surgery while reducing the resulting postoperative adhesions.

Secondly, when? Development of the electromicrosurgery technique was started by the author in 1960, more than thirty years ago. This technique is still useful and provides better results than in-vitro fertilization / embryo transfer (IVF/ET) in suitable patients.

Thirdly, how? Electromicrosurgery incorporates the surgical principle of **"pelvic gentleness"**, that is to say, the surgery is performed as **atraumatically** and as **bloodless** as possible. This can be achieved by utilizing microelectrodes, magnification and good microsurgical principles.

A practical demonstration of the author's technique is shown with four different patients in a 16mm film. This film is available from The Institute for Scientific Film, Göttingen, Germany (film no. C-1469)(Swolin, 1983).

From 1940 to 1964, at the Karolinska Hospital in Stockholm, 106 salpingostomies were carried out with disastrous results, one live birth among those 106 patients (Özaras, 1968). During that period, the Karolinska Hospital was regarded as having the leading gynecology clinic in Sweden and the head of the department was an internationally known infertility expert. Moreover, the diagnostic radiologist Özaras (Özaras, 1968) questioned the value of the infertility surgery available at that time.

However, during the late fifties, intense studies of the literature in the field combined with numerous visits to leading clinics on the European continent provided the author with the possibility of assembling and developing relevant ideas. From these ideas developed the practical applications which are known, today, as the **Microsurgical Principles in Gynecology.** The author had realized that, different from other surgical specialities, one, if not the main, problem in the surgical treatment of gynecological infertility was the development of postoperative adhesions. Consequently, all of the work of the author became focussed on the **goal of preventing adhesions.**

By the beginning of the sixties, the author had developed this work into a personal microsurgical technique. This technique simply incorporated the concept of carrying out the surgery in the most atraumatic and bloodless way possible.

The literature of that time exhibited varying methods for avoiding postoperative adhesions. The results of routine surgery were objectively evaluated by **second-look laparoscopy** in patients being treated surgically for ectopic pregnancy. It was evident that, after such routine gynecological surgery in the small pelvis, **85% of patients developed adhesions** (Swolin, 1967). The literature revealed many more-or-less successful reports on how to reduce adhesions. However, the author concentrated his efforts to some specific techniques: electromicrosurgery, resection of the omentum, the use of heparin and cortisone, and the separation of surfaces with liquids or emulsions. At a later date, the author used, instead of resection of the omentum, a simpler and less bloody method, that is, simple or double plication of the omentum using coarse sutures in order to withdraw it from the small pelvis. Furthermore, there was evidence in the literature that use of the cold knife resulted in more adhesions after surgery compared with thermocautery.

In the opinion of the author, apart from incision of the skin, the entire operation should be performed using **electrosurgery.** For this reason, the author introduced, apart from the presently well-known microsurgical principles, the **microelectrode** into gynecology. In addition, the author is one of a number of surgeons that now believe that the laser is not superior to the microelectrode. For example, the work of Tulandi confirms this opinion (Tulandi, 1984).

According to the traditional teachings of surgical techniques, instruments should be used rather than fingers. However, in microsurgery, **fingers** are regarded as **softer** and **less traumatic** than the surgical instruments.

Magnification is, of course, a basic element of microsurgery but one should be aware of bloody surgery, that is, "butchery under the microscope". A training course in microsurgical technique does not make a good microsurgeon in real life. **Pelvic gentleness** is one of the secrets of excellent microsurgery in gynecology, not only in regard to post-operative function but even in regard to adhesions.

The author also believes in the beneficial effects of **intraperitoneal application of cortisone** for the reduction of adhesions (Swolin, 1966a,b) and has used large doses in his infertility surgery (Swolin, 1968).

As a part of the microsurgical principles, the utilisation of the **wet-chamber technique** during the entire operation also helps to reduce adhesions, since they are also provoked by drying of the serosal surface, Additionally, **non-woven material** is recommended by the author instead of the normal cotton surgical towels. A study by the author has shown that towels of non-woven material are less traumatic to the peritoneum than cotton towels (Swolin *et al*, 1974). Sturdy and coworkers (Sturdy *et al*, 1966) have demonstrated the presence of cotton fibres in microscopic analyses of postoperative granulomas. The **meticulous lavage** at the end of every microsurgery for infertility is essential for the removal of all foreign material, besides the elimination of blood, and blood- and cell-products, such as lysosomes, oxygen-free radicals, etc.

The author would like to emphasize that **early postoperative laparoscopy** is a necessary tool for counteracting postoperative adhesions. In 1975, a demand for this was published in a work on long term results of salpingostomy (Swolin, 1975).

Not the best but reasonable results of good microsurgery are at least 20% live-births after salpingostomy, 60% after lysis of adhesions, and 80% after anastomosis of previous tubal sterilization (Swolin, 1984). In comparison, The American Fertility Association reported in January, 1991, an overall live delivery rate of 14% for IVF in the USA in patients with a tubal disease problem.

Finally, the author believes that there is still a place for excellent microsurgery despite all the advances of assisted reproduction.

The verbal presentation of the above was followed by the film on **Electromicrosurgery in Gynecology, Swolin-technique** (Swolin, 1983).

References:

Özaras, H. (1968) The value of plastic operations on the Fallopian tubes. Acta Obstet. Gynecol. Scand.**47**:489-492.

Sturdy, J. et al. (1966) Surgical sponges: A cause of granuloma and adhesion formation. Ann. Surg. **165**:128-134.

Swolin, K. (1966a) Resection of the Fallopian tubes in the monkey with and without large doses of glucocorticoid. Acta Obstet. Gynecol. **45**:451-472.

Swolin, K. (1966b) Experimental studies on the profylaxis of intraperitoneal adhesions.Studies in the rat with an emulsion of lipid and prednisolone. Acta Obstet. Gynecol. Scand. **45**:473-498.

Swolin, K. (1967) The influence of large intraperitoneal doses of glucocorticoid on the development of postoperative adhesions. Clinical studies by laparoscopy on patients operated for ectopic pregnancy. Acta Obstet. Gynec. Scand.**46**:204-216.

Swolin, K. (1968) Fifty fertility operations, I. Literature and methods. Obstet. Gynecol. Survey **23**:382-396.

Swolin, K. et al. (1974) Traumatization of the abdominal serosa. A comparison between non-woven and cotton abdominal swabs. Acta Chir. Scand. **140**:203-204.

Swolin, K. (1975) Electromicrosurgery and salpingostomy. Long term results. Am. J. Obstet. Gynecol. **121**:418-419.

Swolin, K. (1983) Elektro-Mikro-Chirurgie, Swolintechnik in der Gynäkologie. Film C-1469, Institut für den Wissenschaftlichen Film, Nonnenstieg 72, D-3400, Göttingen, Germany.

Swolin, K. (1984) Possibilities of reconstructive tubal surgery. Wien. Med. Wochenschrift **134**:393-396.

Tulandi, T. (1984) Reconstructive surgery of hydrosalpinx with and without the carbon dioxide laser. Fertil. Steril. **42**:839-842.

Gynecologic Surgery and Adhesion Prevention, pages 51–58

ADHESION FORMATION AFTER LAPAROSCOPY

Annette I. La Morte
Michael P. Diamond
Department of Obstetrics and Gynecology
Yale University School of Medicine
333 Cedar Street
New Haven, Connecticut 06510

Laparoscopic pelvic surgery is becoming increasingly popular. When compared to traditional surgical methods, laparoscopy has many advantages. These include decreased hospitalization time and decreased postoperative pain. A reduction in postoperative adhesion formation is felt by some to also be an important benefit of laparoscopic surgery. However, this view is supported primarily by anecdotal evidence, personal expectations, or eternal optimism. Because adhesion formation is felt to adversely affect fertility, surgical techniques resulting in decreased postoperative adhesion development are of prime importance in the gynecologic armamentarium.

Estimations regarding the incidence of adhesion formation after laparotomy are varied. Earlier reports have reported postoperative adhesions in 55-100% of patients following reproductive pelvic surgery at laparotomy (Surrey & Friedman, 1982; Daniell & Pittaway, 1983; Diamond et al, 1984; DeCherney & Meyer, 1984; Pittaway et al, 1985; and Trimbos-Kemper et al, 1985). These numbers include de novo adhesion formation which has been reported to be as high as 51% of women (Diamond et al, 1987). Adhesion reformation after microlaser techniques during laparotomy have occurred in 40% to 72% of patients (McLaughlin, 1983).

Clinical studies examining adhesion formation and reformation post-laparoscopy have been limited. There has been no study comparing adhesion formation following laparoscopy and laparotomy in the same clinical trial where similar procedures were performed and similar techniques used. Animal studies may be better controlled, but results cannot be directly extended to the human population.

In spite of these limitations, a number of investigations have attempted to clarify the incidence of adhesion formation following laparoscopic pelvic surgery in both animals and humans. This review summarizes the available literature on this topic.

Two well-controlled animal studies comparing adhesion formation after laparoscopy and laparotomy showed conflicting results. Filmar et al in 1987 used a rat model to study adhesion formation after a standard tissue injury (Filmar et al, 1987). Sixty-one white female rats were divided into two groups. One group of rats underwent a 10-15 minute laparoscopic procedure. Three superficial cuts using sharp scissors were made on the antimesenteric surface of the left uterine horn. The cuts involved the serosa and the superficial muscularis. The second group of rats had an identical tissue injury performed during a 10-minute laparotomy. A second-look laparotomy was performed on all rats. The majority of rats in each group had adhesion formation to the site of injury. There were no adhesions on the uninjured uterine horn. The total area involved in adhesions was compared between groups. The laparoscopy group had a higher mean area, but the difference was not statistically significant. One problem with this study is that bleeding was noted to occur from the area of injury in all instances in the laparoscopy group with no reference made to controlling hemostasis.

Luciano et al in 1989 published a study comparing postoperative adhesion formation following a laser injury by laparoscopy versus laparotomy (Luciano et al, 1989). Twenty female white rabbits were divided into equal groups. One group underwent laparoscopy with laser ablation of the antimesenteric wall of the uterine horn and ablation of a 2 cm^2 peritoneal surface of the lower abdominal wall. The second group of rabbits had similar laser injuries produced during laparotomy. Three weeks after the initial procedure a second-look was performed. No adhesions were seen in the post-laparoscopy group. All rabbits post-laparotomy had adhesions at the operative sites and some had de novo adhesions (formed at non-operative sites) in addition. The group with adhesions had laser adhesiolysis carried out via laparoscopy in 5 animals and via laparotomy in the other 5 animals. Autopsies were performed 3 weeks later. The mean postoperative adhesion scores were similar between the two groups. The laser laparoscopy group, by chance, started with a higher adhesion score prior to adhesiolysis and showed a significant decrease in adhesion score. There was no change in adhesion score in the laser laparotomy group. The authors concluded that the number of adhesions that developed postoperatively were significantly greater when the operative procedure was performed by laparotomy rather than laparoscopy. Furthermore, laparotomy was associated with the formation of de novo adhesions and laser laparoscopic adhesiolysis was effective in reducing adhesions.

Seven uncontrolled clinical studies have examined adhesion formation and reformation post-laparoscopy. Nezhat et al in 1990 reported on adhesion reformation after laser laparoscopy for the treatment of endometriosis-associated infertility (Nezhat et al, 1990). No sutures or medical adjuvants were used. One hundred and fifty-seven patients underwent a second-look laparoscopy 4-18 months after their initial surgery. Second-looks were performed because of persistent infertility, recurrence of pelvic pain, ectopic pregnancy, or electively at the time of D&C for spontaneous abortion. Seven sites were assessed for adhesion reformation, including both ovaries and tubes, omentum/bowel, and anterior and posterior cul-de-sac. Adhesion scores were assessed retrospectively by a single observer reviewing the videotaped procedures. A standardized scoring system of 0 to 3 was used. At second-look laparoscopy, no de novo adhesions were present. A significant reduction in the mean postoperative adhesion scores at each of the study sites was observed and an overall 60-79% reduction in adhesions at all sites was observed.

The Operative Laparoscopy Study Group (1991) assessed adhesion reformation following laparoscopic adhesiolysis in a multi-center study (Diamond et al, 1991). Sixty-eight patients underwent operative laparoscopy, including adhesiolysis. A variety of modalities were used, including laser, electrocautery, and sharp dissection. No medical adjuvants were used at the end of the initial procedures. Second-look procedures were performed within 90 days of the initial procedures. At both procedures adhesions were graded at 9 sites, including both ovaries and tubes, omentum, cul-de-sac, pelvic sidewall, large bowel and small bowel. Adhesions were scored on a scale of 0 to 3. At the time of second-look, adhesion scores were decreased in 86.8% of women, and by an average of 52%. However, postoperative adhesion reformation occurred in 97.1% of women, and 11.8% of patients developed de novo adhesions.

Redwine (1991) examined the difference in adhesion scores at initial laparoscopy and at second-look surgery in women treated for endometriosis. Eighty-one women underwent laparoscopy with complete sharp excision of endometriosis and adhesiolysis by the same surgeon. A minority of the patients were treated with Interceed as an adhesion barrier after this compound became available towards the end of the study period. Reoperations were performed by the initial surgeon in 48 of the cases and by other surgeons in 33 cases. At reoperation, 40% of patients had an unchanged adhesion score. The adhesion score was decreased in 16% and increased in 44%. Adhesions were seen in 37% of patients at initial surgery and 60% at reoperation. The time intervals from the initial to the second surgery ranged from less than 3 months to 6 1/2 years, with 50% of the reoperations performed prior to 15 months from initial surgery.

Fayez et al in 1991 reported on adhesion formation and reformation after laparoscopic treatment of ovarian endometriomas. One hundred and twenty-four women were randomized into one of four treatment groups. The first group was treated by excision of their endometriomas. The second group was treated by drainage and stripping of the endometrioma lining. The third group underwent drainage with laser vaporization of the endometrioma lining, and the fourth group had simple drainage of the endometrioma. All procedures were performed by the same surgeon. No sutures were used. All patients had 750 ml of Ringer's lactate left in the pelvic cavity and all patients were treated with post-operative danazol. A second-look laparoscopy was performed 8 weeks after the initial surgery. The percent of women in each group with adhesions at second-look were 100%, 37%, 30%, and 27% in groups 1 through 4, respectively. Only group 1 with 35% adhesions initially showed a statistically significant difference between percent of adhesions at initial surgery and at second-look.

Gürgan et al in 1991 examined adhesion formation following laparoscopic ovarian electrocautery or ovarian Nd:YAG laser photocoagulation of polycystic ovaries. Seventeen patients were divided into the two treatment method groups. Heparinized Ringer's lactate was left in the pelvis after the initial procedure. Second-look laparoscopy was performed 3 to 4 weeks after the initial laparoscopic intervention. Eighty-two percent of patients had periovarian adhesions at second-look. The majority of adhesions were minimal to mild.

Dunn (1991) examined 11 patients at second-look laparoscopy 12 to 21 days following laser laparoscopic adhesiolysis. No intraoperative agents were used for adhesion prevention. Fifteen sites were evaluated for adhesions. All patients had adhesion reformation in at least one site. Fifty-six percent of available sites had adhesions at second-look laparoscopy, which was not a significant change from the 60% of sites with adhesions at initial laparoscopy. De novo adhesions formed in 7 of the patients at 23% of available sites.

Nezhat et al (1991) assessed adhesion formation following laparoscopic myomectomy with and without suture-closure of the defect. Fifty-six patients underwent a second-look procedure between 2 and 24 months following surgery. Overall, 53% of patients had adhesions at reoperation. Of the 37 patients where no suture was used, 24% had adhesion formation. Of the 19 patients who had suture used, 100% had adhesion formation.

In summary, postoperative adhesion reformation following laparoscopic pelvic surgery appears to be similar to that seen following surgical procedures performed at the time of laparotomy. The incidence of de novo adhesions does seem to be decreased following laparoscopic surgery, with the two larger studies (Nezhat et al, 1990 and Diamond et al, 1991) reporting 0% and 12% of patients with de novo adhesion at second-look procedures. However, appropriately controlled clinical trials are needed before a reduction in postoperative adhesion formation can be definitively listed as an advantage of laparoscopy over laparotomy.

Importantly, we must also be sure that when terms such as "adhesion reformation" or "de novo adhesion formation" are utilized, that all reports are describing the same process under the same conditions. Unfortunately, this has not always been the case; when Diamond et al (1991) discussed "de novo adhesion formation," they were referring to development of adhesions at sites which did not undergo adhesiolysis at the time of the initial surgical procedure. In contrast, when Nezhat et al (1990) described "de novo adhesion formation," they referred to sites which did not undergo adhesiolysis, and additionally, were not operated upon at the initial surgery. Thus, the definition of the same term has had different meanings. To minimize this confusion, and to allow comparison of "apples with apples" and oranges with oranges," we would like to suggest the following adhesion classification system based on the presentation given at the Second International Symposium on Gynecologic Surgery and Adhesion Prevention (Diamond, 1992):

POSTOPERATIVE ADHESION DEVELOPMENT

Type 1) De novo adhesion formation - Development of adhesions at sites which did not have adhesions initially.
- a. No operative procedure at site of adhesion formation.
- b. Operative procedure performed at site of adhesion formation.

Type 2) Redevelopment of adhesions at sites at which adhesiolysis was performed.
- a. No operative procedure at site of adhesion formation (other than adhesiolysis).
- b. Operative procedure performed at site of adhesion reformation (in addition to adhesiolysis).

REFERENCES

Daniell JF, Pittaway DE (1983): Short-interval second-look laparoscopy after infertility surgery: a preliminary report. J Reprod Med 28:281.

DeCherney AH, Mezer HC (1984): The nature of posttuboplasty pelvic adhesions as determined by early and late laparoscopy. Fertil Steril 41:643.

Diamond MP (1992): Laparoscopic surgery. Second International Symposium on Gynecologic Surgery and Adhesion Prevention, Palm Beach, Florida, January, 1992.

Diamond MP, Daniell JF, Feste J, McLaughlin DS, Martin DC (1984): Pelvic adhesions at early second-look laparoscopy following carbon dioxide laser surgery procedures. Infertility 7:39.

Diamond MP, Daniell JF, Feste J, Surrey MW, McLaughlin DS, Friedman S, Vaughn WK, Martin DC (1987): Adhesion reformation and de novo adhesion formation after reproductive pelvic surgery. Fertil Steril 47:864.

Diamond MP, Daniell JF, Johns DA, Everett R, Hill GA, Reich H, Martin DC, Maxson WS, Hoffman DI, Murphy AA, Feste J (Operative Laparoscopy Study Group) (1991): Postoperative adhesion development after operative laparoscopy: evaluation at early second-look procedures. Fertil Steril 55:700.

Dunn RC (1991): A longitudinal, observational study of adhesion reformation and de novo adhesion formation after laparoscopic adhesiolysis. (Abstr. 0-013) Presented at the 47th Annual Meeting of The American Fertility Society, Orlando, Florida, October 21-24, 1991. In the Program Supplement, Published by the American Fertility Society, Birmingham, Alabama, p S6.

Fayez JA, Vogel MF (1991): Comparison of different treatment methods of endometriomas by laparoscopy. Obstet Gynecol 78:660.

Filmar S, Gomel V, McComb PF (1987): Operative laparoscopy versus open abdominal surgery: a comparative study on postoperative adhesion formation in the rat model. Fertil Steril 48:486.

Güran T, Kisnisci H, Yarali H, Develioglu O, Zeyneloglu H, Aksu T (1991): Evaluation of adhesion formation after laparoscopic treatment of polycystic ovarian disease. Fertil Steril 56:1176.

Luciano AA, Maier DB, Koch EI, Nulsen JC, Whitmn GF (1989): A comparative study of postoperative adhesions following laser surgery by laparoscopy versus laparotomy in the rabbit model. Obstet Gynecol 74:220.

McLaughlin DS (1983): Evaluation of adhesion reformation by early second-look laparoscopy following microlaser ovarian wedge resection. Fertil Steril 42:531.

Nezhat CR, Nezhat FR, Metzger DA, Luciano AA (1990): Adhesion reformation after reproductive surgery by videolaseroscopy. Fertil Steril 53:1008.

Nezhat C, Nezhat F, Winer W, Evans D (1991): Postoperative adhesion formation after laparoscopic myomectomy with and without suturing. (Abstr. 0-110) Presented at the 47th Annual Meeting of The American Fertility Society, Orlando, Florida, October 21-14, 1991. In the Program Supplement,

Published by the American Fertility Society, Birmingham, Alabama, p S48.

Pittaway DE, Daniell JF, Maxson WS (1985): Ovarian surgery in an infertility patient as an indication for a short-interval second-look laparoscopy: a preliminary study. Fertil Steril 44:611.

Redwine DB (1991): Conservative laparoscopic excision of endometriosis by sharp dissection: life table analysis of reoperation and persistent or recurrent disease. Fertil Steril 56:628.

Surrey MW, Friedman S (1982): Second-look laparoscopy after reconstructive pelvic surgery for infertility. J Reprod Med 27:658.

Trimbos-Kemper TCM, Trimbos JB, van Hall EV (1985): Adhesion formation after tubal surgery: results of the eighth-day laparoscopy in 188 patients. Fertil Steril 43:395.

Gynecologic Surgery and Adhesion Prevention, pages 59–63

TECHNIQUES IN LAPAROSCOPY THAT REDUCE POSTSURGICAL ADHESIONS

James F. Daniell, M.D.
Bryan R. Kurtz, M.D.
Centennial Medical Center
Nashville, Tennessee 37203

INTRODUCTION

The explosion in endoscopy, spurred on by the growth in laparoscopic procedures being performed by the general surgeons, has pushed the gynecologist to look at alternatives to conventional laparotomy in increasing frequency. More and more procedures are being performed laparoscopically, offering the patients the benefit of minimally invasive surgery with its reduced hospital costs and quicker recovery time.

One of the biggest concerns of any type of surgery is the risk to the patient of postoperative adhesions. After major abdominal pelvic surgery, as many as 60-80% of patients will have postoperative adhesions.[1] This risk is especially significant in infertility surgery. Studies have shown that from 55-100% of patients undergoing reproductive pelvic surgery by laparotomy will have subsequent postoperative adhesions diagnosed by early second-look laparoscopy.[2-8] This includes not only adhesion reformation, but also de novo adhesion formation.

Adhesion prevention at laparoscopy is a very complicated and significant problem. Many adjuvants have been tried in the past, but none have really proven efficacious. Barrier methods of protection have included INTERCEED and Gortex mesh.[9-11] The problem with INTERCEED placement is that the tissue must be dry for placement, and it must be free of any ooze or bleeding. Our experiences with INTERCEED at laparoscopy have also included judicious use of early second-look laparoscopy. It is our opinion that INTERCEED works only in situations in which it can be applied to a dependent area in the pelvis, and that most likely, when applied around the tube or ovary, it probably falls off very rapidly. Gortex also can be difficult to place, as it requires securing with suture or staples. Furthermore, being non-absorbable limits the application around the ovary or tube.

Recently, interest has focused on newer solutions that may reduce adhesions, including sodium hyaluronate and a liquid form of tolmetin.[12,13] Other earlier used substances such as intraperitoneal steroids and high molecular weight Dextran has now been discarded, based on data suggesting that they are not efficacious and have never been approved for general use.[14] We have been involved in preclinical trial evaluations of both sodium hyaluronate and tolmetin at laparoscopy. These studies have included operative laparoscopy followed by the pouring into the peritoneal cavity through the laparoscopic trocar of a liquid solution of either of the two substances or a saline study solution. Second-look laparoscopy a month later has been used to assess postoperative adhesion or readhesion formation. To date, the efficacy of these two investigative products is unknown, as a multi-center prospective double blind study is in progress.

The organ that unfortunately attracts the greatest amount of adhesions is the ovary, and in our opinion, there is no effective method of significantly reducing ovarian adhesion formation when any sort of ovarian trauma occurs at laparoscopic surgery. Various methods of laparoscopic surgery have been used over the last decade, including cautery and laser energy of various types, including CO_2, Nd:YAG, argon, and KTP lasers. In our decade's experience with these various laser modalities, we have seen significant adhesions at second look in many patients, no matter what type of laser energy is used.

It is our opinion that the most efficacious method of reducing postsurgical adhesions is to limit the trauma at the time of the initial operative procedure. No matter what type of method is used, tissue handling should be meticulous, irrigation should be copious, and residual clot and fibrin should be minimized. All separated adhesions should be removed meticulously if possible, and there should be no bleeding in the pelvis at the end of the procedure. At present, our regime involves copious irrigation with heparinized Ringers (5,000 units in 1 liter) with 200-300 cc of heparinized Ringers being left at the end of the procedure, unless INTERCEED or a Gortex patch has been placed. We then offer selected patients an early second-look laparoscopy, particularly in those cases in which ovarian or tubal surgery has been performed.

Recently, new mechanical devices have become available for laparoscopic surgery that produce less trauma. These include the automatic stapling devices and use of permanent laparoscopic clips, both absorbable and non-absorbable. In addition, smaller sutures can now be used via laparoscopy with small microinstruments and with more advanced suturing techniques. These techniques allow reduction in intraoperative trauma and at early followup, appear to reduce postsurgical adhesions.

LAPAROSCOPIC STAPLING DEVICES

The new laparoscopic stapling devices, although expensive, allow automatic stapling and transection of tissue for advanced pelviscopic procedures. We have used these extensively for laparoscopic assisted vaginal hysterectomy, appendectomy, and oophorectomy.[16-18] In addition, laparoscopic assisted vaginal hysterectomy can now be performed usually as a one-day or overnight stay procedure, allowing more rapid recuperation from this type of procedure for patients.

Laparoscopic clip appliers now are available in both reusable and disposable preloaded clip handles. The advent of laparoscopic clips now allows one to accomplish more effective hemostasis without the trauma associated with excessive use of cautery or lasers of various types for hemostasis. The permanent titanium staples appear to be nonreactive, based on long term evaluation in other surgical specialties such as pulmonary and GI surgery. Reabsorbable staples are being evaluated, but as of this writing, there is not significant data on postoperative adhesion formation following the absorbable staples. In our practice, we use laparoscopic staples made of titanium in situations in which we want to approximate raw surface edges, (e.g. after presacral neurectomy) or to close large ovarian defects after ovarian surgery, or for hemostasis in areas in which we would be afraid to use sutures, cautery, or laser energy (for example, close to bowel serosa or the ureter). Just as clips have been of tremendous value in the past at laparotomy for hemostasis near vital structures, they can now be applied laparoscopically when indicated with excellent hemostasis and with minimal risk of lateral trauma to adjacent structures.

USE OF THE ARGON BEAM COAGULATOR

It is now possible to use unipolar cautery in a non-touch technique at laparoscopy. This is a very new modality we have been exploring for about a year in our practice.[19] The argon beam coagulator was approved for laparoscopic surgery in the fall of 1991 after extensive preclinical trials. The manufacturer (Birtcher Medical) has now developed 10 and 5 mm probes for laparoscopic delivery of the argon beam coagulator. The argon beam coagulator allows unipolar coagulation in a non-touch technique. A needle electrode which is recessed inside a laparoscopic probe is activated, and the energy from the needle electrode is carried through space through a small plume of high flow (4 liters/min.) argon gas. This argon gas captures electrons from the needle electrode, and then energy is carried through space to impact on the tissue. The bolus of argon gas blows any oxygen in the peritoneal cavity away from the impact site, reducing smoke production. The tissue plume also blows debris and blood away from oozing sites so that the coagulation effect is directly on the bleeding tissue. This gives less depth of penetration and more rapid, effective coagulation at laparoscopy. The spot size at present with this probe is 3 mm, which means that tissue effect is not at a fine point, so this can not be used for fine delicate surgery. It does, however, allow effective rapid hemostasis in a smokeless environment, and in our experience has been very effective for hemostasis for laparoscopic myomectomy, ectopic pregnancy, adhesiolysis, uterosacral ligament transection, and particularly for laparoscopic coagulation of endometriosis.

Biopsy of the argon beam coagulator impact sites indicate histology exactly the same as other unipolar cautery sites, except depth of penetration is usually not more than 2-3 mm.[20] At open surgery, urologists have used this on the ureter and bladder, and general surgeons have used it on the bowel serosa. Our experience at open surgery has found this to be an effective, rapid method for dissecting near the bowel and ureter. Thus we have been able to accomplish effective laparoscopic surgery while reducing the costs associated with laser surgery while also reducing our operating times because of the lack of smoke with the ABC.

There are potential complications that might occur from argon beam coagulator use through the laparoscope. These include the possibility of embolism of argon gas because of the high flow rates that occur, and accidental overdistention of the patient from failure to vent off the high inflow of argon gas. The technology is very inexpensive compared to lasers, with the top-end argon beam coagulator for laparoscopy, which also includes a unit for bipolar and unipolar coagulation, costing under $15,000.00. Laparoscopic probes for the argon beam coagulator are disposable, but are much less expensive than laser fibers.

EARLY SECOND-LOOK LAPAROSCOPY TO REDUCE ADHESIONS

In our professional opinion, the most efficacious method of reducing postsurgical adhesions is the judicious use of early second-look laparoscopy. In our experience, adhesions become dense and vascularized within 6-8 weeks after initial lysis with either open or laparoscopic techniques. Thus, early second-look laparoscopy at 3-6 weeks gives a window of opportunity, when results of the initial surgery can be accurately assessed and gentle lysis with aquadisection and blunt probing can usually be carried out. Second-look laparoscopy sooner than 3 weeks usually results in the tissue bleeding from residual edema, and later than 6 weeks usually finds dense fibrotic adhesions that require extensive operative procedures at the second look. The use of second-look laparoscopy after infertility surgery has been well established following laparotomy, and now has been recommended and used by many investigators after laparoscopic surgery.[15] This is actually the only way that one can accurately assess the early postoperative effectiveness of therapeutic modalities at the initial laparoscopic procedure.

Early data does now indicate that adhesions do form after laparoscopic lysis.[15] However, these adhesions are not as dense as those occurring after laparotomy and are easier to lyse than adhesions seen at laparotomy. In addition, the incidence of de novo adhesions is less at second-look laparoscopy after laparoscopic surgery.

CONCLUSIONS

We are entering an exciting era in endoscopic surgery in which more and more information is becoming available about adhesion prevention and possible adjuvant therapy for adhesion reduction at laparoscopy. In addition, new technology is becoming available that allows more aggressive procedures to be performed with less trauma to tissue. In this era of cost containment, it behooves all of us to investigate all methodology that might allow us to more effectively perform minimally invasive surgery. As technology improves and equipment changes, we should all look carefully at all new items that come down the pike and try to determine whether they may play an effective role in successful laparoscopic surgery.

REFERENCES

1. Weibel MA, Majno G (1973): Peritoneal adhesions and their relation to abdominal surgery. Am J Surg 126:345-353.
2. Diamond MP (1988): Gynecology and Obstetrics, Vol. 5 In Sciarra JJ (ed): "Surgical Aspects of Infertility." Philadelphia: Harper and Row, p 1.
3. Surrey MW, Friedman S (1982): Second-look laparoscopy after reconstructive pelvic surgery for infertility. J Reprod Med 27:658-660.
4. Daniell JF, Pittaway DE (1983): Short-interval second-look laparoscopy after infertility surgery: a preliminary report. J Reprod Med 28:281-283.
5. Diamond MP, Daniell JF, Feste J, McLaughlin DS, Martin DC (1984): Pelvic adhesions at early second look laparoscopy following carbon dioxide laser surgery procedures. Infertility 7:39-44.
6. DeCherney AH, Mezer HC (1984): The nature of posttuboplasty pelvic adhesions as determined by early and late laparoscopy. Fertil Steril 41:643-646.
7. Pittaway DE, Daniell JF, Maxson WS (1985): Ovarian surgery in an infertility patient as an indication for a short-interval second-look laparoscopy: a preliminary study. Fertil Steril 44:611-614.
8. Trimbos-Kemper TCM, Trimbos JB, van Hall EV (1985): Adhesion formation after tubal surgery: results of the eighth-day laparoscopy in 188 patients. Feril Steril 43:395-400.
9. Linsky CB, Diamond MP, Cunningham TJ, et al (1987): Adhesion reduction in the uterine horn model using an absorbable barrier, TC7. J Reprod Med 32:17-20.
10. Interceed (TC7) Adhesion Barrier Study Group (1989): Prevention of postsurgical adhesions by Interceed (TC7), an absorbable adhesion barrier: a prospective, randomized multicenter clinical study. Fertil Steril 51:933-938.
11. Boyers SP, Diamond MP, DeCherney AH (1988): Reduction of postoperative pelvic adhesions in the rabit with Gore-Tex surgical membrane. Fertil Steril 49:1066-1070.
12. Urman B, Gomel V (1991): Effect of hyaluronic acid on postoperative intraperitoneal adhesion formation and reformation in the rat model. Fertil Steril 56:568-570.
13. Rodgers KE, Girgis W, Johns D, et al (1989): Intraperitoneal tolmetin prevents postsurgical adhesion formation in rabbits. Int J Infertil 34:40-45.
14. Jansen RPS (1985): Failure of intraperitoneal adjuncts to improve the outcome of pelvic operations in young women. Am J Ostet Gynecol 153:363-371.
15. Operative Laparoscopy Study Group (1991): Postoperative adhesion development after operative laparoscopy: evaluation at early second-look procedures. Fertil Steril 55:700-704.
16. Daniell JF, Gurley LD, Kurtz BR, Chambers JF (1991): The use of an automatic stapling device for laparoscopic appendectomy. Obstet Gynecol 78:721-723.
17. Daniell JF, Kurtz BR, McTavish G, Gurley LD, et al (1991): Laparoscopic assisted vaginal hysterectomy: the initial Nashville experience. J Reprd Med (submitted)
18. Daniell JF, Kurtz BR, Lee JY (1991): Laparoscopic oophorectomy: comparative study of ligatures, bipolar coagulation and automatic stapling devices. (in press)
19. Daniell JF, Fisher B, Alexander W (1991): Laparoscopic evaluation of the argon beam coagulator: initial report. J Reprod Med (in press).
20. Brand E, Pearlman N (1990): Electrosurgical debulking of ovarian cancer: a new technique using the argon beam coagulator. Gynecol Oncol 39:115-118.

Gynecologic Surgery and Adhesion Prevention, pages 65–80

IMPACT OF LASERS ON POST-OPERATIVE ADHESIONS

Jacques Barbot, M.D.
Hôpital St. Jacques
Paris, France

Our subject raises a number of issues which together form the outline of the study. If we admit, as it seems logical to do, that post-operative adhesions are related to the trauma caused by the surgical procedure itself, we can assume that the ideal surgical tool is one which best preserves tissue integrity. In practice, there are three available techniques. First of all, sharp instruments which act solely by contact without any diffusion. They best preserve adjacent tissues. Unfortunately, the necessity of hemostasis most often requires the use of sutures or coagulation. Thus this advantage is lost. Electrosurgery allows both cutting and hemostasis at the cost of cellular damage over an area of variable size which is difficult to control. The use of microelectrodes or bi-polar forceps tends to limit the diffusion area. The laser is the only instrument which can act upon the tissue without coming into contact with it. Its tissue effects vary widely according to the type of laser used and the expertise of the surgeon in handling the operating parameters. Proper use requires good understanding of the nature of laser energy and its action. We will begin by recalling the basic concepts. The choice of the type of laser used is a very sensitive point given the cost of investment. No one laser has all the qualities, thus a compromise must be found. The CO2 laser will be our reference. Its tissue effects have been widely studied and its features combine precision, safety, minimal tissue damage and excellent healing. Logically it should give rise to few post-operative adhesions. Unfortunately it is poorly adapted to endoscopy which is increasingly used. Other types of lasers having the advantage of fiberoptic transmission are becoming more popular. None is equal to the CO_2 laser as regards tissue sparing. Their value lies more in their ease of use in endoscopy and in some selective effects. Two questions should be answered with regard to post-operative adhesions. Does laser surgery result in fewer postoperative adhesions than surgery performed with sharp instruments or electrosurgery? Of all available lasers, which one creates the least adhesions?

Comparative studies can be performed on animal models, providing for better quantification of parameters than in the human. However it is difficult to extrapolate their results to human beings. Hence the need for clinical studies. It may be tempting to assess postoperative adhesions indirectly, for instance by the pregnancy rate after infertility surgery. But there are too many factors involved for the analysis to be fully convincing. Postoperative laparoscopic assessment is more objective. Direct viewing of adhesions is not subject to doubt. This is the method we have adopted to compare the results of the CO_2 laser versus electrosurgery following infertility surgery. As techniques evolve rapidly, new fiber-transmitted lasers are under experimentation. Their effects are drawing closer to those of their CO_2 counterparts.

Recent data tend to demonstrate that operative laparoscopy yields fewer adhesions than intraabdominal surgery. This should not modify the results of comparative studies performed using conventional surgery and assessed by second look laparoscopy as regards the amount of adhesions which can be attributed to each technique, laser or electrosurgery.

The Nature of Laser Energy

The laser beam is an electromagnetic radiation similar to natural light which we are very accustomed to. However, its mode of creation which is based on stimulated emission endows it with new properties which are potentially contained in natural light, but which cannot express themselves because of its incoherent mode of production. On the other hand, stimulated emission makes it possible to produce a coherent light beam, i.e. one whose waves are spacially and temporally in phase. These beams which are pure in frequency and only slightly divergent convey highly concentrated light energy. It is the interaction between this light energy and living tissue which is the basis of laser surgery.

Interaction of Laser Energy with Living Tissue

Laser/ tissue interaction is extremely complex depending both on the physical parameters of the incident radiation and on the characteristics of the living tissue target. Radiation parameters involve wavelength, power output, beam diameter and delivery mode. Tissue reaction is affected by many factors, such as chemical composition, color, density, local vasculature, thermal conductivity, absorption and scattering coefficients. Such an interaction results in various effects including thermal effects due to absorption of radiant energy and conversion into heat, photochemical effects related to selective absorption by one chemical component, electrical effects due to interaction with the electromagnetic field of the radiation and mechanical effects produced by accoustic shock waves. In fact only the thermal effect is commonly used in gynecology to obtain cutting, vaporisation or coagulation effects, in the absence of which no laser energy would exist.

Thermal Effects of the CO2 Laser

Most studies concerning adhesion formation and their recurrence have been carried out using the CO2 laser which is still by far the most frequently used laser in gynecology. The CO2 laser is a gas molecular laser that emits light in the infrared range. The main feature of the 10.6 micron wavelength generated by the CO2 laser is to be intensely absorbed by water. Living soft tissues being mainly composed of water, the laser/tissue interaction results essentially in a thermal effect and this effect is not color-dependent. The 10.6 radiation is also heavily absorbed by glass and this precludes its transmission through a standard quartz optical fiber.

The incident laser beam striking the surface of the laser target undergoes three effects which are: reflection upon the interface, absorption and scattering within the tissue.

The reflection upon the interface of the CO2 laser beam is usually low and not color dependent. The energy which has not been reflected back interacts within a volume of tissue (the impact or interactive volume) whose dimensions depend on the value of the scattering and absorption coefficients.
Scattering results in a loss of power density by enlargement of the interactive volume and dilution of the energy. It is wavelength dependent and negligable in the case of the CO2 laser while it is important in the case of the Nd:YAG laser. (1.06 micron)

Absorption turns radiant energy into heat. A high absorption coefficient means low depth of penetration. In the case of the CO2 laser, 99.9% of the energy is absorbed within a depth of 0.1 mm. The Yag laser, whose absorption coefficient is low, allows penetration into tissues 10 to 15 times deeper. Low penetration depth and low scattering result in small interactive volume containing a high power density which allows rapid rise in temperature until the boiling point of 100° celsius is reached causing cells to explode under the pressure of the steam and debris to be burnt in the ambient air.

This ability to remove matter through vaporization accounts for the excellent tissue cutting and ablation performance of the CO2 laser. On the periphery of the interactive volume site, heat is carried away as a function of thermal condictivity and blood convection of tissue and temperature decreases. Proteins are coagulated when a temperature of 60°C, which is the threshold for protein denaturation, is reached. This provides hemostasis which is very pleasant for the operator, but also tissue necrosis, which is less welcome when a cutting effect is desired. However, this outer fringe of thermal damage is minimal because of the excellent efficiency of the conversion of radiant energy to heat which allows very short exposure times. For this reason, healthy tissue adjacent to the laser incision is spared, but hemostatic achievement is poor, only affecting vessels not larger than 0.5 mm in diameter. On the contrary, the Yag laser creates a very large interactive volume in which coagulation and necrosis prevail.

Practical Use of CO2 Laser

It appears that the major factor of laser/tissue interaction is power density, i.e. the energy delivered per time unit to an area unit of tissue, practically expressed in joules per second (or watts) per square centimeter. The operator can adjust at will the power output, the diameter of the beam (spot size) and the duration of exposure to obtain various effects.

- The power output is selected on the control panel
- Spot size depends on the focal length of the lens used to focus the beam at the end of the articulated arm. Handpieces allow shorter focal distance than microscopes and therefore smaller spot sizes (0.1 mm in diameter for a focal length of 5 cm). The operator can enlarge the spot size by defocussing. It suffices to move the focal point a little bit away from the tissue surface. This maneuver is far more efficient than altering the power output when a change in power density is needed.
- Laser exposure time can be preset on the console and activated by pressing on a foot pedal or control by the operator by moving the beam across the tissue more or less rapidly.
- The cutting effect will be obtained by focussing the beam and moving it along the incision line.

The ablation of a mass of tissue requires a larger spot size which is obtained by defocussing the beam or by using a lens with a longer focal length. In both cases, the mass of tissue which is a function of the amount of energy (the power x time product) which is delivered. By contrast, the extent of coagulation necrosis depends almost exclusively upon the time of exposure. Given a precise dose of energy, it is advisable to use the combination of a high wattage and short exposure duration to minimize the outer fringe of thermal damage.

The conflicting requirements of operating precision and minimal tissue necrosis have led to the development of the "super pulse" technique of laser energy delivery. Brief pulses of high power are separated by a pause allowing the resulting average power to reconcile slow operating velocity with short exposure duration.

Hemostasis is obtained by defocussing the beam until the power density becomes too low to vaporize tissue and causes only coagulation necrosis.

Tissue carbonization is the result of a faulty technique (use of a low power density with excessive time on tissue). It is damaging because carbonic residues absorb heat and increase tissue temperature unnecessarily.

Problems Raised by the Adaptation of the CO2 Laser to Endoscopic Surgery

The wavelength of 10.6 microns produced by the CO2 laser is strongly absorbed by glass. This prohibits its delivery through conventional fiberoptics. To get around this problem the beam has to be transmitted through the air by means of a hollow articulated arm provided with mirrors which bend the beam. This arm ends with a handpiece equipped with a focussing lens. Though it is acceptable for intraabdominal surgery, this articulated arm is very cumbersome for endoscopic surgery. Furthermore, the laser beam must be focussed through a sleeve inserted through the abdominal wall. This requires the use of a longer focal distance lens and thus increases spot size. Alignment along the firing axis is also more delicate. The wave guide has a smaller diameter tube and solves the problem of spot alignment. However, it must always be connected to the articulated arm.

True fiberoptics capable of transmitting the CO2 laser beam are still experimental and none to date has the qualities of conventional flexible quartz fiberoptics.

Lasers transmitted by Conventional Quartz Fiberoptics

Nd:YAG Laser

The amplifying medium is no longer a gas but a crystallin solid instead which emits in the near infrared red at 1.06 micron. This wavelength is easily transmitted by quartz in the form of optical fibers 200-600 microns in diameter. The laser beam loses its coherence after passing through the fiber. This has only limited consequences for laser surgery using only the thermal effect. Moreover, when leaving the fiber the beam diverges by roughly 10 to 15°. The smallest spot size is obtained when the fiber is in contact with the tissue and then is equal to the diameter of the fiber.

The Nd:YAG laser tissue effects are very different from those of its CO2 counterpart. The YAG laser beam is only slightly absorbed by water in tissue resulting in penetration 10 to 15 times greater. Scattering off the direction of the forward beam becomes important. Interactive volume is increased, energy is diluted and the efficiency of heat conversion is reduced. The increase in temperature is slower and rarely reaches 100° C, required to vaporize cellular water. The result is a large volume of extensive thermal necrosis, but a poor cutting effect. Forward scattering displaces into the tissue the point of maximal power density making the produced effect more unpredictable and less controlable.

Argon and KTP/532 Lasers

The argon laser is a gas laser emitting in the visible blue-green spectrum (488 to 514.4 nm). The KTP/532 laser is a Nd:YAG rod combined with a potassium titanyl phosphate crystal producing harmonics among which the Nd:YAG wavelength (1064 nm) is frequency doubled (532 nm) and extracted. Its wavelength is close to the argon laser and its effects in tissue are similar. The only advantage is a gain in power when compared to the argon laser whose output is limited. The effect on tissue of these two lasers is highly color dependent. Their rays are not strongly absorbed or scattered by water and colorless tissue. Consequently they can penetrate deeply into non-pigmented tissue with little scattering. On the contrary, they are strongly absorbed by reddish tissue containing hemoglobine or melanin. The KTP 532 laser achieves enough power density to vaporize these tissues, but coagulates only small volumes because of the low amount of scatter. On the whole, they do not cut or vaporize as well as the CO2 laser nor coagulate as well as the Nd:YAG laser and they cause an intermediate amount of tissue damage.

Nd:YAG Laser Emitting at a Wavelength of 1.32 Microns

The Nd:YAG laser which is currently used in surgery is designed to emit at a wavelength of 1.06 microns. However, its crystal has other transitions ranging from 0.939 μ to 1.44 μ. Some of them can be amplified to the detriment of 1.06 μ albeit with a loss of efficiency. It's possible to amplify the 1.32 μ transition.

This wavelength is particularly interesting as the water absorption curve versus wavelength reveals a sharp increase when going from 1.06 to 1.32. This means better efficiency of the conversion into heat and tissue effects which are closer to those of the CO2 laser. Several studies of the tissue effects at this wavelength have been performed on the animal model. The results confirm theoretical expectations. For the same penetration, less energy is required at 1.32 μ wavelength than at 1.06 μ. This means shorter exposure time and consequently lesser thermal damage. A lower scattering coefficient also contributes to obtain a clear cut and a smaller coagulation fringe.
The 1.32 Nd:YAG laser has been clinically used with success for several years in neurosurgery. Its action on brain tissue provides vaporization close to the CO2 laser and similar tissue damage. Hemostasis is comparable to that of the conventional Nd:YAG laser. In gynecological surgery,

we have been using for three years a MC 2100 laser (Technomed, France) which can emit either at 1.06 or 1.32 μ. Switching from one setting to the other can be done immediately on the control panel. The superpulsed mode further reduces the fringe of thermal damage. Delivery is realized by conventional quartz fiberoptics 200-600 microns in diameter. During laparoscopy, there is less plume release than with the CO2 laser. The more pale the tissue is, the better the cutting effect will be. It allows the removal of ovarian cysts and of myomas, adhesiolysis and salpingostomy.

Assessment of Postoperative Adhesion Formation in the Animal Model

The complexity and the great number of factors interfering with postoperative adhesion formation in a clinical situation and the difficulties raised by proper control and valid interpretation of the results in evaluating new techniques has led to the use of animal models which, theoretically, are simpler. The animal model has numerous advantages. The selection of the best experimental design and its achievement are not hampered by the usual ethical problems specific to the human. Proper randomization and control groups can be easily obtained among a population which is supposed to be homogeneous. The parameters of the experiment can be precisely quantified and reproduced and the number of variables is limited. Randomized and comparable subgroups allow to carry out comparative studies concerning the effectiveness of various techniques and therapeutic tools. The control can be immediate for evaluation of the acute tissue damage or at various periods after surgery for long term assessment of chronic tissue damage and adhesion formation.

However, the animal model has disadvantages and limitations. Despite the attempt the obtain an animal population which is homogeneous, within the same species wide variations in the individual response have been noted in several studies, especialy concerning adhesion formation. Consequently, only a subgroup including a large number of animals can provide valid data for statistical analysis and this requirement is not always fulfilled in some studies, making their conclusions doubtful.

But the major disadvantage with animal studies is that their results cannot be extrapolated with certainty to the human. No matter how closely the animal model mimics a clinical situation, the extrapolation remains questionable in the finally analysis, it is impossible to elude clinical studies.

In the past ten years, many animal studies have been devoted to the evaluation of the laser as a surgical tool opposed to the more conventional techniques using sharp instruments or electrocautery. Most of them were comparative studies dealing with the CO2 laser versus electrosurgery as regards tissue damage and adhesion formation. With the increasing development of operative laparoscopy, more recent studies have assessed the value of new lasers delivered through a fiber and compared open surgery with laparoscopic surgery.

Some of the early comparative reports involving the CO2 laser were conflicting. However, with a heightened understanding of the relation between power density and thermal injury and the greater regard given to proper statistical analysis, a consensus seems to be emerging from the latest studies.

We reviewed 18 studies published between 1981 and 1991 dealing with the impact of lasers on tissue damage and postoperative adhesions in the animal model. This review is not, of course, exhaustive but it provides a fair understanding of the surgeons' concern and the way in which they tackle these problems has changed over the years.

The rat model was chosen in 6 studies and the rabbit model in 12 studies. The number of animals included in each study ranged from 4 to 61 in the rat and from 5 to 40 in the rabbit. In the 14 comparative studies, the subgroups ranged from 4 to 31 specimens in the rat model and from 5 to 40 specimens in the rabbit model. Randomization is mentioned in 6 reports and the same animals were assigned to a control group or served as their own control in 6 experiments. Acute or chronic tissue damage was histologically evaluated in 12 studies and adhesion formation was evaluated in 14 studies. The effectiveness of the CO2 laser was assessed in 14 studies using a conventional articulated arm in 12 cases but a superpulsed model was tested in 2 cases. Concerning the more recent lasers which are delivered through a fiber, the Nd:YAG laser with a sapphire tip was used in 3 experiments, the argon laser was tested in one study and the KTP/532 in another study.

Among the latest lasers tested in gynecology, the Er:YAG laser and the Ho:YAG laser were included in one comparative study.

The comparative studies opposed the conventional CO2 laser to electrosurgery in 5 cases and to both sharp instruments and electrosurgery in 2 cases. The CO2 laser was also opposed to the Nd:YAG laser and electrosurgery in another experiment. The CO2 laser in a supersulsed mode was tested against sharp instruments in one case and against the CO2 laser in a continuous mode in another case. Finally, one study compared postoperative adhesion formation following the use of scalpel, electrocautery, Nd:YAG laser, Er:YAG laser and Ho:YAG laser. Concerning tissue damage, out of 5 studies opposing the CO2 laser to electrosurgry, one study found that the CO2 laser caused less injury than electrosurgery, one study yielded opposite results and no significant difference was demonstrated in 3 other experiments. It must be pointed out that the 2 conflicting experiments used either a very small number of animals or an early type of laser producing a low power density and a large spot size. In the supersulsed mode, the CO2 laser appeared to provide better tissue healing than sharp instruments in one experiment and less thermal necrosis than the CO2 laser in a continuous wave mode in another

comparative study. The Nd:YAG laser with a sapphire tip was found to provoke significantly greated thermal injury than the CO2 laser or electrosurgery in one experiment.
Concerning postoperative adhesion formation, 11 comparative studies involving the use of various lasers were available. 8 experiments compared the effect of the CO2 laser used in a continuous wave mode with more traditional techniques using sharp instruments and electrosurgery. Six of them did not achieve any significant difference and two of them found an advantage in the use of the laser. However, one of them was stastistically criticizable. The superpulsed CO2 laser was tested against the continuous wave CO2 laser in one study and the adhesive response appeared to be significantly diminished in the pulsed-treated group. Five studies evaluated the effectiveness of the CO2 laser and the Nd:YAG laser with a sapphire tip in adhesiolysis and demonstrated no statistically significant difference in the two modalities. In the same way, 2 studies failed to achieve significant difference when opposing the Nd:YAG laser and electrosurgery. One recent experiment comparing YAG lasers using various active media (neodymium, holmium or erbium, rare earth ions) found that the Ho:YAG laser produced less adhesion and the Er:YAG more adhesion than the now classical Nd:YAG laser.

If we exclude some early studies performed with lasers now considered as obsolete or providing inadequate data for statistical analysis, more consistent conclusions can be drawn from this review. The extent of thermal damage caused by the continuous mode CO2 laser is not significantly different from that caused by electrosurgery. The superpulsed CO2 laser appears to provoke less damage than the continuous wave CO2 laser but its effect was not widely tested. Even with a sapphire tip, the Nd:YAG laser causes more thermal damage than the CO2 laser or electrosurgery. As for the argon laser and the KTP/532, they were not included in a comparative study.
Concerning the extent of postoperative adhesions and the effectiveness of adhesiolysis, no significant difference is demonstrated when using electrosurgery. continuous wave CO2 laser or Nd:YAG laser with a sapphire tip. Surprisingly, although the Nd:YAG laser is associated with more thermal tissue damage, this does not seem to result in a greater rate of postoperative adhesions. The Ho:YAG laser is promising but needs further investigation.

Clinical Assessment of Postoperative Adhesion Formation

The assessment of postoperative adhesion formation may be achieved in different ways. When pelvic pain appears to be related to pelvic adhesions and motivates a surgical procedure, subsequent symptomatic improvement may be interpreted as a sign of non-recurrence of the disease. However, many factors, in particular of a psychological nature, may influence the results and no definitive conclusions can be inferred.
In the case of infertility associated with periadnexal

adhesions pregnancy outcome following adhesiolysis may also be considered as an indirect sign of the absence of adhesion reformation. But we know that the adhesive status of the pelvis is only one among many factors that affect pregnancy outcome and it is difficult to evaluate the weight of one individual factor within an overall result.
By allowing direct vision of the pelvis, second look laparoscopy is undoubtedly the most accurate method for objectively detecting the presence of adhesions and for assessing the results of a surgical procedure as regards their formation or recurrence.
Questionable when performed solely for this purpose, there are other advantages which justify it, the main one being to possibility to correct and improve the results for the first procedure by separating the newly-formed adhesions. Another advantage is to provide a prognosis which without any further delay can promote another option such as IVF in the case of discouraging results.

The timing of this second look procedure is subject to discussion. In our personal practice we perform second look laparoscopy 8 days after the initial procedure. One advantage is its good acceptance by patients in so far as it is performed just before dismissal from hospital. Furthermore, adhesiolysis, when required, is easier to perform when the adhesions are freshly reformed, causing only loose attachments between the anatomic structures. Simple pressure or traction is often sufficient to bluntly separate the surfaces in contact without causing bleeding. One could object that the readhesion process is not completed 8 days postoperatively but we know that it starts very early, within a few days following surgery and that if the adhesions are not yet organized, they are already present at all sites at that time.

In order to compare the efficacy of the CO_2 laser versus electrosurgery for adhesiolysis we took advantage of our experience with second look laparoscopy that we had been routinely practicing for several years to conduct a comparative study using this procedure as an objective means to assess the rate of adhesion reformation at all sites where adhesiolysis had taken place during intraabdominal infertility surgery.

172 patients having infertility related to tuboperitoneal factors underwent intraabdominal surgery using microsurgical techniques and magnification as provided by the Zeiss OPM 16 micro (Oberkochen, Germany). Our group included 94 patients that had been referred to our center (St. Jacques Hospital, Paris) using the CO_2 laser since 1980 for all infertility surgery and the other group included 78 patients referred to another center (Port Royal Hospital, Paris) using only electrosurgery for the same procedures. With the exception of the "use or non use" of the CO_2 laser, the two centers utilized the same instrumentation, the same operating technique and the surgical teams had the same training with one surgeon being common to the two centers.

The selection of patients and the pre- and postoperative treatments were also similar in the two centers. Although the two groups were not randomized, chance had it that the process of referrals to one center or the other evened out the populations and so the two groups turned out to be comparable. The surgical procedures were carried out simultaneously, during the same period of time in the two centers. All patients had periadnexal adhesions associated in 114 cases with tubal damage (cornual, isthmic, ampullary occlusion or stenosis). Adhesions were assessed and scored using the international classification adopted at the 10th World Congress on Fertility and Sterility (Madrid 1980). Briefly, this classification separates adhesions into type A, thin and scarce; type B, moderate and partially encapsulating; and type C, severe and extensive. Patients having type A adhesions were excluded from this study as we don't perform second look laparoscopy following adhesiolysis in such cases, the results usually being excellent whatever the technique and we consider their influence on pregnancy outcome too low to justify such a procedure.

The laser group used a hand-held Coherent 450 CO2 laser and adhesiolysis was performed in a continuous mode at a mean power density of 2500 w/sq. cm. Except for the unique CO2 laser technique of directly vaporizing the filmy adhesions covering the ovary surface, the adhesions were lysed in a similar manner with the CO2 laseror the microelectrode. Adhesiolysys was performed on 294 adnexa, 136 having adhesions classified as moderate (type B) and 158 having adhesions classified as severe (type C). Postoperative laparoscopy was performed 8 days postoperatively on the 172 patients initially included in this study. There was no exclusion which could have been related to last moment refusal on the part of the patient or from postoperative complications. Recurrent adhesions were scored as present or absent at each site where adhesiolysis had taken place.

The previous classification was not used as the adhesive process is not completed at this early stage and no valid comparison can be made concerning the type of adhesion, all of them appearing viscous and loose. In the case of recurrence, they could be easily separated with minimal bleeding. No complication occured and all the patients were dismised from hospital the next day. We found that when lysis had been performed on adhesions scored as moderate (type B), the recurrence was 15% for all those cases using electrosurgery and 9% when the CO2 laser was used. When lysis was performed on adhesions scored as severe (type C), reformation was recorded in 25% of the electrosurgery treated cases and in 19% of the laser treated cases.

Although the rate of recurrence was lower in the laser group, statistical analysis revealed that the difference was not significant. (p 0.05).

Several remarks can be made in light of this study. The frequency of adhesion reformation after adhesiolysis assessed by second look laparoscopy differs widely from one study to another.

When performing second look laparoscopy 8 days

postoperatively, Kemper et al. demonstrated adhesions in more than 50% of cases. All operations were performed without magnification and with the use of electrocautery. Diamond et al. assessed adhesion reformation after operative laparoscopy by performing a second look procedure within 90 days. Adhesion recurrence was found in 66 of 68 women. In this multicenter study, various instruments were used for adhesiolysis (sharp dissection, electrocoagulation, CO2 laser, argon laser, KTP laser) and no comparison was made between the different techniques.
Using the CO2 laser for laparoscopic adhesiolysis in 157 patients, Nezhat et al. found at late second look laparoscopy that adhesions were reduced by 60 to 79% at all sites without the formation of new adhesions.
Garrel performed second look laparoscopy on ten patients who failed to conceive after laparoscopic salpingo-ovariollysis using scissors. No residual adhesive process was seen. Our study was designed to assess adhesion reformation at the site of adhesiolysis 8 days after intraabdominal surgery. The maximal rate of recurrence was 25%.
These variations are probably related to a lack of homogeneity between the different studies as regards the number of surgeons involved in each case, the scoring of lesions, the instrumentation and technique used for adhesiolysis and the timing of the second look procedure.

Concerning the efficacy of the CO2 laser versus electrosurgery, the results are more consistent. In our study no statistical difference was reached concerning the rate of recurrence of postoperative adhesions and this is in agreement with the results found in animal studies.
In a multicenter prospective study assessing the results of adhesiolysis by means of second look laparoscopy performed within 12 weeks of the intraabdominal procedure, Diamond et al. achieved no surgical difference in the prevention of adhesions.
If we now consider the pregnancy rate after adhesiolysis performed either with electrosurgery or with the CO2 laser, the same conclusions can be drawn. Comparing salpingo-ovariolysis performed with each technique in a randomized prospective trial, Turlandi et al. found no statistical difference in the pregnancy rate. The same author condusted a similar study for bilateral hydrosalphinx and no significant difference could be demonstrated. When using the CO2 laser for laparoscopic adhesiolysis in 59 patients, Donnez achieved a pregnancy rate of 57%, similar to that obtained after microsurgical lysis by laparotomy.
In fact, the pregnancy rate achieved after salpingo-ovariolysis in the absence of tubal damage in most studies ranges from 50 to 60%, irrespective of the technique and instrumentation used. When we know that adhesion reformation is a major factor in failures following infertility surgery, a rate of success of 50% or more proves that adhesiolysis is effective and we must not adopt too pessimistic a view concerning adhesion reformation in spite of the high incidence of recurrence found in some studies.

Use of Fiber Delivered Lasers

These lasers are increasingly used for laparoscopic surgery. Several studies report on there use with or without sapphire tips for photovaporization of endometriosis (argon or KTP/532 laser), removal of ovariancysts, adhesiolysis or salpingostomy. Results seem satisfactory however, to date as far as we know, no clinical comparative study is available concerning postoperative adhesions. When we performed second look laparoscopy after using the 1.32 μ YAG laser we observed a low rate of adhesion but we do not have enough cases to draw valid conclusions. Comparative studies in the animal model using those lasers have demonstrated that all caused more thermal damage than the CO_2 laser. It is also unlikely that they cause less adhesion. However it seems that more thermal tissue damage does not always imply more postoperative adhesions. This point calls for more study. The advantage drawn from greater ease of use and consequently from shorter operating time must be weighed against slightly greater thermal damage.

Conclusion

The impact of the laser on postoperative adhesions has been mainly assessed with regard to the CO_2 laser. Most comparative studies performed in the animal model as well as in the clinical setting tend to prove that it is not superior to electrosurgery as regards postoperative adhesion formation. Concerning the fiber delivered laser, we are lacking comparative studies assessing the incidence of postoperative adhesions. Theoretical considerations based on tissue effects lead us to believe that they are not superior to the CO_2 laser in this field.
However, these results do not forbid the use of lasers in infertility surgery in so far as they do not create more adhesions than electrosurgery. Each type of laser in its own field has specific advantages (non-contact surgery, hemostasis, selective destruction of peritoneal endometriosis, vaporization of ovarian endometriomas, salpingostomy "flowering"). They participate in the advance of gynecological surgery and may make interesting contributions in the future.

REFERENCES

Badawy, SZA et al: Pulsed CO2 Laser Versus Conventional Microsurgical Anastomosis of the Rat Uterine Horn. Fertil Steril 46:127, 1986

Baggish, MS. and Chong, AP.: Carbon Dioxide Laser Microsurgery of the Uterine Tube. Obstet Gynecol 58:110, 1981

Baggish MS and ElBakry, MM: Comparison of Electronically Superpulsed and Continuous-Wave CO2 Laser on the Rat Uterine Horn. Fertil Steril 45:120, 1986

Baggish, MS and ElBakry, MM: A Flexible CO2 Laser Fiber for Operative Laparoscopy. Fertil Steril 46:16, 1986

Baggish, MS et al: Carbon DioxideLaser Laparoscopy by Means of a 3.0-mm Diameter Rigid Wave Guide. Fertil Steril 50:419, 1988

Barbot, J. et al.: A Clinical Study of the CO2 Laser and Electrosurgery for Adhesiolysis in 172 Cases Followed by Early Second-Look Laparoscopy. Fertil Steril 48:140, 1987

Bhatta, N et al: Comparison of Post-Operative Adhesion Formation and Histologic Thermal Damage Following Ovarian Wedge Resection in Rabbits Using Scalpel, Electrocautery, Er:YAG, Nd:YAG or Ho:YAG Laser. 47th Annual Meeting of the American Fertility Society S-48:O111, 1991

Daniell, JF et al.: Initial Evaluation of the Use of the Potassium-Titanyl-Phosphate (KTP/532) Laser in Gynecologic Laparoscopy. Fertil Steril 46:373, 1986

Daniell, JF et al: Laser Laparoscopic Management of Large Endometriomas. Fertil Steril 55:692, 1991

Daniell, JF and Herbert, CM: Laparoscopic Salpingostomy Utilizing the CO2 Laser. Fertil Steril 41:558, 1984

DeCherney, AH and Mezer, HC: The Nature of Posttuboplasty Pelvic Adhesions as Determined by Early and Late Laparoscopy. Fertil Steril 41:643, 1984

Diamond, M. et al: Postoperative Adhesion Development After Operative Laparoscopy:Evaluation at Early Second-Look Procedures. Fertil Steril 55:700, 1991

Diamond, MP et al: Adhesion Reformation and De Novo Adhesion Formation After Reproductive Pelvic Surgery. Fertil Steril 47:864, 1987

Diamond, MP et al: Tubal Patency and Pelvic Adhesions at Early Second-Look Laparoscopy Following Intraabdominal Use of the Carbon Dioxide Laser: Initial Report of the Intraabdominal Study Group. Fertil Steril 42:717, 1984

Donnez, J.: CO2 Laser Laparoscopy in Infertile Women with Endometriosis and Women with Adnexal Adhesions Fertil Steril 48:390, 1987

Fayez, JA et al: Comparison of Tubal Surgery with the CO2 Laser and the Unipolar Microelectrode. Fertil Steril 40:476, 1983

Filmar, S et al.: Operative Laparoscopy versus Open Abdominal Surgery: a Comparative Study on Postoperative Adhesion Formation in the Rat Model. Fertil Steril 48:486, 1987

Filmar, S et al: The Effectiveness of CO2 Laser and

Electromicrosurgery in Adhesiolysis: a Comparative Study. Fertil Steril 45:47, 1986

Frishman, GN et al: A Comparative Analysis of Adhesion Reduction, Tissue Effects and Incising Characteristics of Electrosurgery, CO2 Laser and Nd:Yag Laser at Operative Laparoscopy. 47th Annual Meeting of the American Fertility Society S-48:0-112, 1991

Gomel, V: Salpingo-Ovariolysis by Laparoscopy in Infertility. Fertil Steril 40:607, 1983

Keye, WR et al: Argon Laser Therapy of Endometriosis: A Review of 92 Consecutive Patients. Fertil Steril. 47:208, 1987

Keye, WR et al: The Use of the Argon Laser in the Treatment of Experimental Endometriosis. Fertil Steril 39:26, 1983

Luciano, AA et al: Ovarian Function After Incision of the Ovary by Scalpel, CO2 Laser and Microelectrode. Fertil Steril 56:349, 1991

Luciano, AA et al: A Comparison of Thermal Injury, Healing Patterns and Postoperative Adhesion Formation Following CO2 Laser and Electromicrosurgery. Fertil Steril 48:1025, 1987

Luciano AA et al: A Comparative Study of Postoperative Adhesions Following Laser Surgery by Laparoscopy Versus Laparotomy in the Rabbit Model. Obstet Gynecol 74:220, 1989

Lundorff, P et al: Second Look Laparoscopy After Ectopic Pregnancy. Fertil Steril 53:604, 1990

Lundorff, P et al: Adhesion Formation After Laparoscopic Surgery in Tubal Pregnancy: a Randomized Trial Versus Laparotomy. Fertil Steril 55:911 1991

Mc Laughlin, DS: Evaluation of Adhesion Reformation by Early Second-Look Laparoscopy Following Microlaser Ovarian Wedge Resection. Fertil Steril 42:531, 1984

Nezhat, C et al: Videolaseroscopy for the Treatment of Endometriosis Associated with Infertility. Fertil Steril 51:237, 1989

Nezhat, C et al: Surgical Treatment of Endometriosis via Laser Laparoscopy. Fertil Steril 45:778, 1986

Nezhat, CR et al: Adhesion Reformation after Reproductive Surgery by Videolaserscopy. Fertil Steril 53:1008 1990

Pittaway, D et al: Ovarian Surgery in an Infertility Patient as an Indication for a Short-Interval Second-Look Laparoscopy: a Preliminary Study. Fertil Steril 44:611, 1985

Pittaway, D et al: A Comparison of the CO2 Laser and

Electrocautery on Postoperative Intraperitoneal Adhesion Formation in Rabbits. Fertil Steril 40:366, 1983

Trimbos-Kemper, TCM et al.: Adhesion Formation After Tubal Surgery: Results of the Eighth-Day Laparoscopy in 188 Patients. Fertil Steril 43:395, 1985

Tulandi, T and Vilos, GA: A Comparison Between Laser Surgery and Electrolsurgery for Bilateral Hydrosalpinx: a Two-Year Follow-Up. Fertil Steril 44:846, 1985

Tulandi, T: Salpingo-Ovariolysis: a Comparison Between Laser Surgery and Electrosurgery. Fertil Steril 45:489, 1986

Wallwiener, D et al: Application du Laser Néodym Yag dans l'adhésiolyse. Rev Fr Gynécol Obstet 11:721 1989

Gynecologic Surgery and Adhesion Prevention, pages 81–95

OVERVIEW OF CLASSICAL ADJUVANT APPROACHES

Gary Holtz, M.D.
Southeastern Fertility Center
Mt. Pleasant, South Carolina 29464

During the early nineteenth century, infectious peritonitis was established to be a causative factor for peritoneal adhesion formation. Subsequently, traumatic, thermal and chemical injuries were also recognized. In 1859, the first therapeutic procedure for symptoms caused by peritoneal adhesions was undertaken, lysis of adhesions for bowel obstruction. Shortly thereafter it became evident that despite meticulous surgical technique, peritoneal adhesion formation, and particularly reformation after lysis, was a major problem for patients undergoing intra-abdominal surgical procedures. As early as 1880, ancillary therapeutic measures were being considered. Although many of the early reports were anecdotal, well designed animal studies with second look procedures allowing asessment of efficacy were also reported (Boys, 1942). Current investigators, therefore, have received a great legacy and one which is too often ignored.

ANTI-BACTERIAL THERAPY

Among the earliest ancillary therapeutic measures were efforts to prevent post-operative bacterial peritonitis. These included adoption of aseptic technique, bacteriophage therapy, and chemotherapeutic measures. Bacteriophage therapy consisted of introducing killed organisms into the peritoneal cavity on the premise that this would induce phagocytosis. Colibactragen was utilized clinically as late as 1940. The development of sulfonamide compounds, and subsequently penicillin, caused the abandonment of these efforts. A survey of reproductive surgeons performed in 1984 revealed prophylactic antibiotics were administered to virtually all women undergoing reproductive pelvic surgery (Holtz, 1985). Dosage programs administered were often therapeutic rather than prophylactic in nature.

MECHANISTIC THERAPY

Many of the early efforts at adhesion prophylaxis were mechanistic. Membranes or sheets of a variety of materials were placed between areas judged to be at risk for adhesion formation/reformation. Many of these materials actually induced severe foreign body reactions with adhesion formation being the consequence. Some of the earliest materials evaluated, such as fetal membranes, continue to be of interest to some investigators (Young, et al, 1991). Similarly, a variety of solutions were instilled into the abdominal cavity as lubricants. Among these were mineral oil, olive oil and vitreous of calves eye. These also were often associated with foreign body reactions. The introduction of crystalloid solutions was common; hypertonic solutions were frequently employed in efforts to induce a further influx of fluid into the abdominal cavity. Although safe, absorption occurred very rapidly, limiting efficacy. One of the more interesting approaches to mechanical separation of injured peritoneal surfaces was the post-operative establishment of a pneumoperitoneum; there is at least one report of clinical application. Clearly this approach, separating peritoneal surfaces, has attracted considerable interest in the last two decades and currently enjoys the most widespread application as will be discussed further.

A somewhat different mechanistic approach involved efforts to either actively or passively cause movement of intra-abdominal viscera and thereby prevent prolonged apposition of injured, fibrin covered peritoneal surfaces. Active peristalsis was stimulated by a variety of substances (physostigmine, strychnine, soap suds enemas); this concept was quite popular in both Germany and the United States at the turn of the century. Post-operative abdominal massage was also recommended. More bizarre approaches included positioning a huge suction bell on the abdomen, and the administration of an iron suspension orally with subsequent movement of a large magnet over the abdomen. The latter was reportedly supported by animal experimentation. Interestingly, recent limited data suggests that a reduction in de novo adhesion formation following laparoscopy, as contrasted to that after laparotomy, may be due to earlier ambulation and the resultant movement of intra-abdominal contents (Das, Penney, and Critser, 1990).

Further efforts included altering the post-operative position of patients in bed in an attempt to employ gravity to separate injured surfaces. Post-operative distension of the bladder and of the bowel with bulky enemas were similarly advocated. Intestinal plication was performed not infrequently after bowel obstruction. Uterine or adnexal suspension and omental plication are similar efforts which have been utilized by reproductive surgeons.

FIBRINOLYTIC THERAPY

Efforts to induce increased fibrinolysis also date to before the turn of the century. These attempts initially involved chemical attacks against fibrin. Hypertonic glucose solutions were among those thought to have fibrinolytic activity, although later studies could not confirm this. The digestive tract enzymes pepsin and trypsin were also evaluated; however both are neutralized by antitrypsin normally found in peritoneal transudates and exudates. Papain was subsequently evaluated; studies of this material continued into the 1960's. However, it is also rendered ineffective by antitrypsin. A third approach involved efforts to stimuate intraperitoneal leukocytosis. Such irritating substances as turpentine were administered in animal studies in efforts to stimulate leukocytosis. The use of amniotic fluid was also based on this rationale. Although the latter was innocuous, it was not effective. Studies of true fibrinolytic agents such as streptokinase often met with success. However, cost and risk of hemorrhage precluded clinical studies. The most recent extension of this approach involves the use of tissue-type plasminogen activator.

ANTICOAGULANT THERAPY

Throughout the twentieth century, efforts to prevent coagulation and deposition of fibrin have emerged. Early experiments involved the use of sodium citrate; initial experiments with heparin were reported in 1935. Clinical usage of substantial dosage regimens has been limited, however, due to the well documented risk of intra-abdominal hemorrhage (Boys, 1942). Use in irrigation solutions is common (Holtz, 1985) despite little documentation of efficacy (Jansen, 1988) (Table 1).

Table 1. Solutions employed for intraoperative irrigation in 1984 (n = 134)

Solution	%
Lactated Ringers with Heparin	55%
Saline with Heparin	14%
Lactated Ringers with Heparin and Steroid	10%
Crystralloid only	16%
Other	5%

ANTI-INFLAMMATORY THERAPY

Mechanisms by which adhesion formation may be reduced include: 1) reduction of the initial inflammatory response and subsequent exudate release, 2) inhibition of coagulation, 3) promotion of fibrinolysis, 4) mechanical separation of fibrin-covered surfaces, and 5) inhibition of fibroblastic proliferation. All but the first and last had received great attention by 1950. Corticosteroids were the first drugs widely employed clinically which could impact on adhesion formation through these remaining mechanisms.

Corticosteroids have been thought to have a variety of actions which might impair adhesion development, including: reducing alterations in vascular permeability; stabilizing lysosome membranes, inhibiting the synthesis and release of histamine and other mediators of the inflammatory response (Replogle, Johnson, and Gross, 1966). They have also been reported to inhibit fibroblast migration and proliferation in animal models, but have been reported to stimulate human fibroblast growth (Granat, et al, 1983). Additionally, they may reduce the intrinsic fibrinolytic activity of the peritoneum.

Corticosteroids are frequently administered in conjunction with promethazine, an antihistamine. This H_1 receptor antagonist limits the release of histamine, inhibits permeability alterations induced by this and other mediators, stabilizes lysosome membranes, inhibits proliferation of mast cells and may inhibit fibroplasia. Despite its widespread utilization, no published study has evaluated its effectiveness as the solely used agent. Indirect evidence suggests it may be equally or more effective than corticosteroids (Gazzaniga, et al, 1975).

Numerous laboratory animal studies have suggested that corticosteroids can reduce adhesion formation and reformation if large doses are administered in the immediate perioperative period. The limited number of primate studies published have reported variable results. Liao, et al (1973) reported that methylprednisolone effectively reduced adhesion formation following a bowel injury. Seitz and colleagues (1973) evaluated adhesion reformation after lysis in monkeys treated with low molecular weight dextran, normal saline or dexamethasone/promethazine. Adhesion formation was similar within the three groups. Unfortunately, a pure surgical control was not included. diZerega and Hodgen (1980) found this regimen to be ineffective in reducing adhesion formation after fallopian tube abrasion.

Only two clinical studies have been reported in which second look procedures were consistently performed. Swolin (1967) administered 2000 mg. of hydrocortisone as a single intraperitoneal dose in patients being operated on for ectopic pregnancy. Second look laparoscopies were performed three months later to assess adhesion formation. Patients who received hydrocortisone had significantly less adhesion formation than did controls; however, treatment was not randomized among the surgeons involved, raising the possibility that variation in operating technique was a factor. Jansen (1985) reported that corticosteroid administration failed to have a significant impact on adhesion formation/reformation, however.

Despite the limited clinical documentation of efficacy, widespread usage has occurred. The collaborative study of Horne and colleagues (1973) has often been cited for this popularity. They reported minimal morbidity associated with the use of a dexamethasone/phenergan regimen. This was in contrast to the concerns expressed by Grosfield, et al (1973) about the use of corticosteroids for adhesion prophylaxis in a pediatric surgical population. In a survey of reproductive surgeons conducted in 1979, over half utilized corticosteroid-containing regimens (Pfeffer, 1980). Usage remained common in 1984 as determined by a survey of the members of the Society of Reproductive Surgeons (Holtz, 1985). However, utilization then was often associated with concurrent intraperitoneal administration of high molecular weight dextran solutions.

Side effects associated with their use have been infrequently reported (Table 2). Impaired wound healing is no longer a significant concern in view of the widespread utilization of synthetic absorbable suture materials which exhibit prolonged retention of strength. Similarly, concerns over immunosuppression and an increased incidence of infection have been attenuated by the near universal concurrent prophylactic administration of antibiotics. The mood elevation asociated with their administration has often been considered favorably by surgeons. Post-therapy depression was the most common adverse effect.

Table 2. Number of Respondents who Attributed an Adverse Reaction to the Use of a Corticosteroid Regimen for Adhesion Prophylaxis.

Adverse Reaction	No. of Respondents
Psychiatric Disturbance	15
Malaise/Bone or Muscle pain post-therapy	6
Edema	2
Adrenal Suppression	1
Disseminated Herpes	1
Thrush	1
Wound Separation	1
Bleeding Ulcer	1
Vein Sclerosis	1
Vaginal Burning	1

Nonsteroidal anti-inflammatory drugs (NSAID) have been of interest as ancillary therapy for nearly 40 years. Despite early favorable studies with oxyphenbutazone, little attention was given to this class of drugs until after the report of Siegler, et al (1980) which demonstrated efficacy when utilizing ibuprofen. This delay can be attributed to the unattractive side effective profile of earlier NSAIDs, and to the difficulty of administering oral drugs in animal models. The development of well tolerated, parenteral products was the impetus for additional studies.

These drugs have a variety of actions including inhibition of prostaglandin biosynthesis, platelet aggregation and secretory activity, leukocyte migration and phagocytosis, and suppression of lysosome release (Gernaat and Stubbs, 1980). They may also allow increased macrophage activity and fibrinolytic activity (Rodgers, 1990).

Results of the numerous animal investigations conducted have varied (Holtz, 1984; Rodgers, 1990). They have consistently included preoperative and intra-operative administration of the NSAIDs; however, dosage regimens have varied greatly. The only clinical study initiated was terminated prematurely, presumably because of a lack of apparent efficacy. However, the dosage utilized was low when contrasted to those administered in animal studies which reported efficacy. Despite this, there was limited clinical usage reported in the author's 1984 survey (Holtz, 1985). There remains significant interest in this group of drugs; this is not unexpected in view of the heterogeneous nature of these pharmaceutical products and the widely differing capabilities they exhibit. Moreover, many of the animal studies may have included inappropriate dosage regimens.

PROPHYLAXIS DURING THE LAST DECADE

During the last decade, the use of 32% dextran 70 in dextrose (Hyskon, Pharmacia) was pre-eminent (Holtz, 1985). Its usage represents one of the most recent efforts to employ an intraperitoneal solution for adhesion prevention.

The rate of absorption of any material instilled within the abdominal cavity is dependent upon molecular weight, solubility, ionic charge and concentration. Dextran solutions have been reported to remain within the peritoneal cavity for variable lengths of time depending on the animal model utilized, concentration of the solution, and molecular weight. Ultrasound studies performed in humans found an increase in intra-abdominal fluid volume up to two weeks after dextran administration (deCherney, 1984). Clearly it causes an influx of fluid into the abdominal cavity because of the osmotic gradient produced. Although "hydroflotation", causing the mechanical separation of injured surfaces, is thought to be the predominant mechanism for adhesion prevention, others exist (Table 3).

Table 3. Postulated Mechanisms of Action for Dextran

1. Hydroflotation
2. Structural alteration of fibrin
3. "Siliconizing" effect on damaging surfaces
4. Reduced shedding of plasminogen activator activity
5. Immunosuppression
6. Maintenance of negative electrical charge on serosa repulsing fibrinogen

Hydroflotation seems to be necessary for the reduction of adhesion reformation after lysis. As previously reviewed, small volumes of Hyskon were effective in reducing de novo adhesion formation after a peritoneal injury, but were not effective in preventing reformation after lysis. In contrast, significantly larger doses were noted to be effective in that application (Holtz, 1984). Dextran also alters the structure of fibrin formed in its presence, producing a significantly coarser network of fibrin strands (Tangen, Wik, and Almquist, 1972). The diameter of these is several times that of fibrin strands formed in the absence of dextran. The more loosely packed structure allows access of plasmin and other fibrinolytic enzymes to the interior of the structure, facilitating lysis. These alterations are caused by the physico-chemical properties of dextran and are shared by other macromolecules. Other actions have limited data supporting them.

Small animal laboratory studies have almost universally suggested that Hyskon reduced adhesion development after a peritoneal injury. As previously mentioned, it was substantially less effective in impeding reformation after lysis. In the only subhuman primate study, it was found to reduce adhesion formation (diZerega and Hodgen, 1980). Four clinical studies with second look procedures have evaluated efficacy in the human. As reviewed at the 1989 symposium, two studies were positive (Adhesion Study Group, 1983; Rosenberg and Board, 1984), and two failed to confirm effectiveness (Jansen, 1985; Larsson, et al, 1985).

Theoretical risks associated with the use of dextran solutions include: allergic reactions, fluid imbalance secondary to the intraperitoneal osmotic load, impaired hemostasis, and infection. In actual clinical usage, clinically significant side effects have been infrequent (Table 4). The most commonly reported adverse reaction was labial edema, secondary to extravasation of fluid (Holtz, 1985). This is disconcerting to the patient but generally not uncomfortable. Administration of low molecular weight dextran solutions has been associated with the development of asymptomatic postoperative pleural effusions in humans. However, the incidence of this occurring with Hyskon was low in the surveyed population. Severe allergic reactions represent the greatest risk. Cul-de-sac aspiration of the intra-abdominal instillate and standard medical therapy have been used effectively for treatment (Borten, Seibert, and Taymor, 1983). Conflicting data exists as to whether Hyskon is a good bacterial culture media (Bernstein, et al, 1982; Elkins, et al, 1985). Routine prophylactic antibiotic usage has largely made this a moot question. Clinically significant impairment of hemostasis has not been noted, but use is contraindicated in the presence of active bleeding.

Table 4. Number of respondents who attributed an adverse reaction to the use of intra-peritoneal dextran 70.

Adverse Reaction	No. of Respondents
Labial Edema	19
Anaphylaxis/Shock/DIC	6
Fever of Unknown Origin	4
Ileus	3
Pleural Effusion/Pulmonary Edema	3
Wound Separation	2

CONCLUSIONS

The list of therapeutic modalities considered for adhesion prophylaxis grows ever longer (Table 5), reflecting the importance of the problem and our inability to effectively reduce adhesion formation/reformation. It is likely the quest will continue for sometime to come. Future efforts will benefit from close inspection of those preceeding.

Table 5: Agents evaluated for adhesion prophylaxis listed by predominant mechanism.

Inhibition of inflammatory reaction and/or fibroplasia:

Antihistamines	Corticosteroids	Progestins
Colchicine	Cytotoxic agents	NSAIDs

Inhibit Coagulation:

Citrates	Hiruden	Oxalates
Heparin	Oral Anticoagulants	Peptone

Promote fibrin lysis:

Actase	Hypertonic glucose	Streptodornase
Amniotic fluid	Papain	Streptokinase
Chymotrypsin	Pepsin	Trypsin
Fibrinolysin	Protoporphyrin	Tissue-type plasminogen activator
Hyalunonidase	Sodium Ricinolate	

Mechanical separation:

Albumin	Lanolin
Agar	Metal foils
Aristol	Mineral oil
Bladder strips	Olive oil
Camphorated oil	Oxidized cellulose
Chyle	Paraffin
Collodion	Peritoneum
Crystalloid solution	Pneumoperitoneum
CMC	Polysiloxanes
Dextran	Povidine
Fat	Silk and rubber sheets
Fetal membranes	Teflon
Gelatin	Thermal sensitive polymers
Gelfilm	Vaseline
Gelfoam	Vitreus of calves eyes
Gum Arabic	
Hyluronic acid	

REFERENCES

Adhesion Study Group (1983). Reduction of post-operative pelvic adhesions with intraperitoneal 32% dextran 70. Fertil Steril 40:612-619.

Bernstein J, Mattox JH, Ulrich JA, Messer RH (1982). The potential for bacterial growth with dextran. J Reprod Med 27:77-79.

Borten M, Seibert CP, Taymor ML (1983). Recurrent anaphylactic reaction to intraperitoneal dextran 75 used for prevention of post-surgical adhesions. Obstet Gynecol 61:755-757.

Boys F (1942). The prophylaxis of peritoneal adhesions. Surgery 11:118-168.

Das K, Penney LL, Critser JK (1990). Effects of passive motion and early versus delayed ambulation on adhesion formation in rat uterine surgery. Int J Fertil 35:245-248.

DeCherney AH (1984). Preventing postoperative pelvic adhesions with intraperitoneal treatment. J Reprod Med 29:157-161.

diZerega GS, Hodgen GD (1980). Prevention of postoperative tubal adhesions: Comparative study of commonly used agents. Am J Obstet Gynecol 136:173-178.

Elkins TE, Trenthem L, McNeeley SG, Ling FW. Prewitt J, Homsey CA, Malinak LR (1986). Potential for in vitro growth of common bacteria in solutions of 32% dextran 70 and 1.0% sodium carboxy-methycellulose. Fertil Steril 43:477-478.

Gazzaniga AB, James JM, Shobe JB (1975). Prevention of peritoneal adhesions in the rat. Arch Surg 110:429-432.

Gernaat CM, Stubbs DF (1980). Clinical brochure for investigators studying ibuprofen and myocardial infarction. The Upjohn Company, Kalamazoo, MI.

Granat M, Schenker JS, Mor-Yosef S, Rosenkovitch F, Castellanos RC, Galili U (1983). Effects of dexamethasone on proliferation of autologous fibroblasts and on the immune profile in women undergoing pelvic surgery for infertility. Fertil Steril 39:180-186.

Grosfield JL, Berman IR, Schiller M, Morse TS (1973). Excessive morbidity resulting from the prevention of intestinal adhesions with steroids and antihistamines. J Pediatr Surg 8:221-226.

Holtz G (1984). Prevention and management of peritoneal adhesions. Fertil Steril 41:497-507.

Holtz G (1985). Current use of ancillary modalities for adhesions prevention. Fertil Steril 44:174-176.

Horne RW Jr, Clyman M, DeBrovner C, Griggs G, Kistner R, Kosasa T, Stevenson CS, Taymor M (1973). The prevention of postoperative adhesions following conservative operative treatment for human infertility. Int J Fertil 18:109-115.

Jansen RPS (1985). Failure of intraperitoneal adjuncts to improve the outcome of pelvic operations in young women. Am J Obstet Gyn 153:363-371.

Jansen RPS (1988). Failure of peritoneal irrigation with heparin during pelvic operations upon young women to reduce adhesions. Surg Gynecol Obstet 166:154-160.

Larsson B, Lalos O, Marsk L, Tronstad S-E, Bygdeman M, Pehrson S, Joelsson I (1985). Effect of intraperitoneal instillation of 32% dextran 70 on postoperative adhesion formation after tubal surgery. Acta Gynecol Scand 64:437-441.

Liao S, Svehiro GT, McNamara JJ (1973). Prevention of postoperative intestinal adhesions in primates. Surg Gynecol Obstet 137:816-818.

Pfeffer WH (1980). Adjuvants in tubal surgery. Fertil Steril 33:245-256.

Replogle RL, Johnson R, Gross RE (1966). Prevention of postoperative intestinal adhesions with combined promethazine and dexamethasone therapy: Experimental and clinical studies. Ann Surg 163:580-588.

Rodgers KE (1990). Nonsteroidal anti-inflammatory drugs (NSAIDs) in the treatment of post-surgical adhesion. In diZerega GS, Malinak LR, Diamond MP, Linsky CB (Eds): "Treatment of post-surgical adhesions," New York: Wiley-Liss, pp.

Rosenberg SM, Board JA (1984). High-molecular weight dextran in human infertility surgery. Am J Obstet Gynecol 148:380-385.

Seitz HM, Schenker JG, Epstein S, Garcia C-R, (1973). Postoperative intraperitoneal adhesions: A double blind assessment of their prevention in the monkey. Fertil Steril 24:935-940.

Siegler AM, Kontopoulos V, Wang CE (1980). Prevention of postoperative adhesions in rabbits with ibuprofen, a nonsteroidal anti-inflammatory agent. Fertil Steril 34:46-49.

Swolin K (1967). Die Einwirkung Von Grossen, intraperitonealen Dosen glukokortikoid auf die bildung von postoperativen Adhaesionen. Acta Obstet Gynecol Scand 46:1-15.

Tangen O, Wik KO, Almquist IAM, Arfors KE, Hint HC (1972). Effects of dextran on the structure and plasmin-induced lysis of human fibrin. Thromb Res 1:487-492.

Young RL, Cota J, Zund G, Mason BA, Wheeler JM (1991). The use of an amniotic membrane graft to prevent postoperative adhesions. Fertil Steril 55:624-628.

Gynecologic Surgery and Adhesion Prevention, pages 97–100

PERITONEAL CLOSURE

Ana Griffin, B.S.
L. Russell Malinak, M.D.
Department of Obstetrics and Gynecology
Baylor College of Medicine
Houston, Texas 77030-3498

ABDOMINAL INCISIONS

It is unclear when the concept of peritoneal closure became incorporated into the practice of surgery. Ambrose Pare (1517-1590) and William Halsted (1852-1922) among other leading surgeons recommended closure of the abdominal wall in layers,[1] without citing previous studies or clinical trials. It appears peritoneal closure has been routinely performed and taught on the basis of clinical impression. Throughout the 20th century many surgeons have questioned the necessity of peritoneal closure.

Controlled study in humans was first reported by Ellis in 1977.[2] He found that separate closure of the peritoneum in a randomized population of general surgical patients played no significant role in the healing of the laparotomy wound. In 1990 Hugh, et al.[3] recommended abandoning separate suture of the peritoneum in general surgical patients. Hull and Varner[4] in 1991 found that non-closure of visceral and parietal peritoneum at low transverse cesarean section had no adverse effect in the postoperative period. A 1990 review by Wadstrom and Gerdin[5] found no studies in which an advantage of layered closure had been demonstrated.

It is our current practice to delete anterior peritoneal closure following abdominal hysterectomy. However, we close the mid-portion of the posterior parietal peritoneum if the vaginal cuff remains open.

In a second look laparoscopy study in infertility patients, Tulandi, et al.,[6] found no significant difference in complications, wound healing, and adhesion to the laparotomy incision with or without peritoneal suturing. He studied presence or absence of adhesions to the anterior abdominal wall, but did not report presence or absence of peritubal and periovarian adhesions.

If the peritoneum is not closed there is a potential for ingress of blood and tissue products from the abdominal wall into the pelvis in the immediate post-operative period. Therefore, we empirically close the peritoneum of abdominal incisions to prevent entry of this fibrin-rich material in patients in whom preservation or enhancement of fertility is a goal of the operation. We also close the peritoneum in order to prevent leakage of dextran when this fluid is utilized for reduction of post-operative adhesions.

PERITONEAL DEFECTS

Adhesion formation associated with closure vs. non-closure of denuded parietal peritoneum at sites other than the incision has not been adequately studied in humans. Prevention of post-operative adhesions is particularly important if pelvic surgery is performed for enhancement or preservation of fertility.

Numerous animal studies have documented: 1) that ischemic peritoneal tissues are potent stimuli to adhesion formation,[7] 2) that deperitonization in the absence of inflammation and ischemia is not the main factor in the causation of adhesions,[8] and that deperitonized surfaces tend to heal without adhesions despite an initial, total absence of mesothelium.[9] Closure of peritoneal defects with sutures which create ischemia will result in adhesion formation,[9,10,14] whereas loosely applied sutures may not.[7,9]

Thus, it appears that closure of peritoneal defects under tension or under other conditions which promote ischemia is more likely to result in adhesion formation than leaving the defects open. Whether loose approximation of peritoneal edges with fine sutures of low tissue reactivity, under conditions not likely to promote ischemia, is frequently associated with adhesion formation is unknown. There has not been adequate study in humans to resolve these issues.

Adhesions (72%) occurred in association with peritoneal defects, some of which were left open, representing the control side of a randomized clinical trial evaluating Interceed to prevent adhesions in a lateral pelvic sidewall application.[13]

Therefore, some method should be utilized to reduce the likelihood of adhesions to a deperitonized pelvic surface when compromise of the internal genitalia might result. The current status of barriers to reduce post-operative adhesions will be covered by other authors.

Finally, most peritoneal defects remaining after hysterectomy and oophorectomy need not be closed. Babcock discovered no ill effects in leaving uncovered excised peritoneal areas of the pelvis in humans.[11] Others observed similar results, noting excellent regeneration and minimal adhesions after extirpation of the peritoneum.[8] Ratcliff, et al noted small bowel obstruction secondary to adhesions at the site of reperitonization after total abdominal hysterectomy; they speculated that non-closure of the parietal peritoneum might reduce the incidence of this complication.[15] Trimpi and Bacon noted that denuded areas which result from excising the peritoneum of the abdominal and pelvic cavities lend themselves well to regeneration and natural repair.[12] They concluded that acceptance of deperitonization without peritoneal suturing allows: 1) more freedom in wide removal of peritoneum when necessary, 2) avoiding hazardous displacement of adjacent viscera, 3) elimination of foreign body reaction from extensive suturing, and 4) shortened operative time.

REFERENCES

1. Halsted WS: Surgical Papers by William Stewart Halsted. The Johns Hopkins Press 2:514, 1924
2. Ellis H and Heddle R: Does the peritoneum need to be closed at laparotomy? Br J Surg 64:733, 1977
3. Hugh TB, Nankivell C, Meagher AP, Li B: Is closure of the peritoneal layer necessary in the repair of midline surgical abdominal wounds? World J Surg 14:231, 1990

4. Hull DH and Varner MW: A randomized study of closure of the peritoneum at cesearean delivery. Obstet Gynecol 77:818, 1991

5. Wadstrom J and Gerdin B: Closure of the abdominal wall: How and why? Acta Chir Scand 156:75, 1990

6. Tulandi T, Hum HS, Gelfand MM: Closure of laparotomy incisions with or without peritoneal suturing and second look laparoscopy. Am J Obstet Gynecol 158:536, 1988

7. Buckman RF, Buckman PD, Hufnagel HV, Gerwin AS: A physiologic basis for the adhesion-free healing of deperitonealized surfaces. J Surg Research 21:67, 1976

8. Robbins GF, Brunschwig A, Foote FW: Deperitonealization: Clinical and experimental observations. Ann Surg 130:466, 1949

9. Ellis H: The cause and prevention of postoperative intraperitoneal adhesions. Surg Gyn Ob 133:497, 1971

10. William DC: The peritoneum: A plea for a change in attitude towards this membrane. Br J Surg 42:401, 1953

11. Babcock WW and Bacon HE: The elimination of colostomy in radical treatment of cancer of the large bowel. Penn Med J 46:1143, 1943

12. Trimpi HD, Bacon HE: Clinical and experimental study in denuded surfaces in extensive surgery of the colon and rectum. Am J Surg 84:596, 1952

13. Interceed Adhesion Barrier Study Group: Prevention of postsurgical adhesions by Interceed (TC7) an absorbable adhesion barrier: a prospective, randomized multicenter clinical study. Fertil Steril 51:933, 1989

14. Elkins TE, Stovall TG, Warren J, et al: A histologic evaluation of peritoneal injury and repair: Implications for adhesion formation. Obstet Gynecol 70:225, 1987

15. Ratcliff JB, Kapernick P, Brooks GG, Dunnihoo DR: Small bowel obstruction and previous gynecologic surgery. Southern Med J 76:1349, 1983

Gynecologic Surgery and Adhesion Prevention, pages 101–120

ADHESIONS AND CHRONIC PAIN: AN OVERVIEW OF PAIN AND A DISCUSSION OF ADHESIONS AND PELVIC PAIN

Margaret R. Punch, M.D.
Randy S. Roth, M.D.
Department of Obstetrics and Gynecology (M.R.P.)
Departments of Anesthesiology and Physical Medicine and Rehabilitation (R.S.R.)
University of Michigan Medical Center
Ann Arbor, Michigan 48109

INTRODUCTION

Controversy exists regarding the etiology and treatment of women with chronic pelvic pain (Renaer and Guzonski, 1978). Despite the high prevalence of chronic pain complaints in gynecologic practice (Henker, 1979) the chronic pelvic pain syndrome remains poorly understood (Beard and Pearce, 1989). Complicating the clinical picture is the common observation that many chronic pelvic pain patients will be found, upon careful diagnostic evaluation, to have no apparent pelvic pathology (Renear, 1980). Still other gynecologic patients who undergo laparoscopic examination, and who are not suffering with pain, are often noted to have significant abnormalities (Trimbos et al., 1990). Moreover, the experienced clinician is familiar with the observation that patients with comparable pelvic disease will differ in the severity and character of their pain. For the gynecologist interested in the relationship between pelvic adhesions and chronic pelvic pain, individual differences in pain experience among chronic pelvic pain patients is no less impressive.

In order to better understand the role of pelvic adhesive disease in chronic pelvic pain, it is important to first obtain a better understanding of the physiological and psychological mechanisms underlying pain experience. Once pain physiology and psychology are reviewed, it becomes easier to understand why there is confusion in trying to clearly define pelvic adhesions as a causative factor in chronic pelvic pain. It also becomes easier to interpret studies looking at adhesiolysis in the management of chronic pelvic pain.

PHYSIOLOGICAL BASIS OF PAIN

Many theories have been proposed to explain pain perception. The earliest and perhaps most influential theory of pain, dating from DesCartes (1664) and popular until the nineteenth century, postulates that stimulation of specific pain receptors results in pain intensity directly proportional to the amount of nerve stimulation. Melzack and Wall (1982) note that remnants of this "specificity theory", while empirically refuted decades ago, continue to influence medical texts describing pain mechanisms. In their review of the evolution of pain theory, these authors point out that virtually all previous theories fail to account for important characteristics of clinical pain including the persistence of pain after healing and the influence of psychological factors on pain perception. To address these shortcomings, Melzack and Wall (1965) introduced their famous gate-control theory of pain. While the original model has been reformulated (Wall, 1978) and is not without its critics (Nathan, 1976) it has been widely heralded for its comprehensiveness and heuristic value in advancing our understanding of pain phenomena. Most importantly for the present discussion, it provides a physiological basis for explaining individual differences in pain experience and the only modest correlation observed between pain behavior and physiologic pathology.

It is well known that painful injury or disease produce afferent impulses that are transmitted by small-diameter fibers - the A-delta and C fibers - which enter the dorsal horn of the spinal cord and activate transmission (T) cells which relay these signals to the brain. Fields (1987) describes this process in two stages: 1) <u>transduction</u> whereby pain receptors (nociceptors) are activated by a stimulus and 2) <u>transmission</u> in which neural processes carry nociceptive information via peripheral sensory nerves, relay neurons ascending in the spinal cord to the brainstem and thalamus, and eventually to reciprocal connections between the thalamus and cortex. The dorsal horn serves as the locus for multiple modulating influences on T cell activation originating from both peripheral and higher brain structures. Large fiber stimulation can activate cells in the substantia gelatinosa and thereby inhibit transmission from afferent fibers to T cells (Wall, 1964; Hillman and Wall, 1969). Similarly, activation of cells in both the periaqueductal grey and nucleus raphe magnus are known to produce profound analgesia presumably through the activation of descending pathways which synapse at the dorsal horn and inhibit the access of nociception to T cells (Fields and Busbaum, 1979). In these ways, the dorsal horn functions as a dynamic gating mechanism within which pain modulation can be achieved through input from both peripheral and central pathways.

Melzack and Casey (1968) further observed that output from T cells project to the brain by way of two ascending pathways, via neospinothalamic fibers to the ventrobasal thalamus and somatosensory cortex and via the medial paleospinothalamic tract that communicates with the recticular formation, the medial and intralaminar thalamus and the limbic system. The authors proposed that neospinothalamic projections are primarily responsible for the transmission of <u>sensory-discriminating</u> information regarding pain. They went on to speculate that the paramedial ascending system, in view of its interconnections with reticular and limbic structures, may be primarily concerned with the <u>motivational-affective</u> dimension of pain which characterizes the emotional distress and behavioral avoidance observed among persons in pain. Lastly, they hypothesized that neocortical and higher central nervous system processes, including <u>cognitive</u> variables such as memories and belief systems, exert influence on both of these sensory and affective pain systems. Thus, pain was viewed as a perceptual (rather than sensory) experience in which sensory, affective and cognitive components interact in a complex pattern of physiological and psychological interplay. The traditional and simplistic notion that an individual is a passive observer (and sufferer) of a pain stimulus gave ground to the evidence that the nervous system is equipped with active endogenous pain modulation mechanisms designed to subdue discomfort in the face of nociception.

Parallel with these advances in the neurophysiology of pain have been important breakthroughs on neurochemical substrates of opiate analgesia and endogenous pain control (Watkins and Mayer, 1982). The recent discovery of two amino acid peptides, leu-enkephalin, and met-enkephalin and the more recent isolation of dynorphin and beta-endorphin provide compelling evidence that these opioid peptides play a crucial role in activating endogenous opioid systems (Bonica 1990a). Of particular interest is the rich concentration of these substances in regions of the central nervous system known to be key to pain perception and modulation such as the dorsal horn, periaqueductal grey, nucleus raphe magnus, and hypothalamus (Fields, 1984). Further, the descending pathways to which these structures give rise are primarily monoaminergic and release serotonin and norepinephrine. Accumulating evidence suggests that both serotonin and norepinephrine mediate opiate analgesia and endogenous pain modulation (Bonica, 1990a). This is of particular importance for the clinician because it provides a biochemical explanation for the therapeutic efficacy of tricyclic antidepressants in the treatment of chronic pain (Getto et al., 1987). These psychoactive agents primarily target serotonergic and noradrenergic neurotransmitter systems (Cooper et al., 1982).

Neural transmission of pain has been more systematically studied in the peripheral somatic tissues (e.g., skin and musculoskeletal systems) due, in part, to the rich innervation of the skin and superficial structures and the relative ease with which they can be tested. Unfortunately with regard to the area of visceral pain, which is of particular relevance to discussions of pelvic pain, the neurophysiologic picture is less clear for several reasons. Because visceral pain tends to be difficult to provoke, it is difficult to identify nociceptors and related afferents (Bonica, 1990b). We do know that pelvic organs contain both sympathetic and parasympathetic innervation. Pain emanating from the uterus and fallopian tubes travel via visceral afferents to the lower thoracic and lumbar sympathetic ganglion and enter the spinal cord at levels T10 through L1. In contrast, the cervix is supplied by parasympathetic fibers which conduct along the pudendal nerves and enter the spinal cord at the sacral segments 2, 3, and 4 (Beard and Pearce, 1989). Visceral pain may also be "referred", that is it is appreciated in an area distant from its origin as a result of segmental convergence of multiple primary afferent nerves at single spinal cord segments (Selzer and Spencer, 1969). Clinically, visceral pain is poorly localized and tends to have a more dull, achy character when compared to superficial pain. Precipitators of visceral pain include tension or traction on hollow viscera, stretching of peritoneum ischemia, infection and inflammation (Bonica, 1990b).

These advances in our understanding of the physiological basis of pain have obvious importance for clinical medicine in its efforts to reduce pain and suffering. However, they also have major implications for promoting a modern view of the psychology of pain. The gathering evidence suggests that pain and psychological processes share common neurobiological pathways. For example, the neural structures (e.g. reticular formation, limbic system) which are said to mediate the motivational-affective component of pain have been recognized for some time to be critical determinants of human emotion and behavior (Heilman and Valenstein, 1979). The aforementioned neurotransmitters serotonin and norepinephrine have similarly been recognized to be pivotal for understanding psychiatric illness, particularly depression (Mason, 1984). The speculation by Melzack and Casey (1968) that cognitive factors such as expectancies, personal beliefs, and memories can influence pain perception through communication between cortical and subcortical brain structures is a further example of a link between physiological and psychological pain processes. These findings have led recent investigators concerned with the psychological correlates of pain to broaden their conceptual view beyond purely psychological mechanisms (Blumer and Heilbronn, 1982). What is emerging is a neuropsychological model of pain perception which will undoubtedly expand our understanding of the way in which nociceptive mechanisms and behavior interact in accounting for variability of pain experience.

PSYCHOLOGICAL BASIS OF PAIN

Interest in psychological factors associated with chronic pain has increased during the past two decades (Aronoff, 1985). Chronic pain often persists in the absence of nociceptive input. It may exceed the healing process and, thus, no longer seem to be a result of disease or injury. As a result, it is not surprising that psychological models arose to explain pain behavior. The fact that, over time, many pain patients develop a chronic pain syndrome - severe functional and vocational disability, narcotic dependency, social withdrawal, alteration in family relationships, fatigue, and depression - has only strengthened efforts to address the psychological dimensions of clinical pain. Early work focused on personality structure and psychodynamic processes such as guilt, masochism, and hysterical defense mechanisms to explain pain of presumed psychogenic origin (Engel, 1959; Walters, 1961; Woodforde and Mersky, 1972). More recently psychologists have studied the contribution of learning theory and reinforcement principles in accounting for pain behavior and its related disability (Fordyce, 1976; Keefe and Gil, 1986). The current "cognitive revolution" in psychology (Mahoney, 1977), which imparts a primary role to cognitive style (e.g., beliefs, self-talk, cognitive schema) to understanding human emotion and behavior, has been a particularly valuable paradigm for ascertaining those factors which account for variability in human pain tolerance and for devising therapeutic approaches to pain control (Turk et al., 1983; Turk and Rudy, 1986).

A variety of psychological treatments have been shown effective in the treatment of chronic pain including relaxation therapy, biofeedback (Turner and Chapman, 1982a), hypnosis, behavior therapy, and cognitive behavioral interventions (Turner and Chapman, 1982b). Consistent with the trend toward cognitive models of behavior, there has been growing interest in the role of coping strategies and belief systems as moderators of the correlation between pain and disability. Patients who possess a belief that they can control their pain, who minimize catastrophizing and negative (e.g. distorting) perceptions and who believe they can function even with pain exhibit better adjustment to chronic pain (Jensen et al., 1991). Of particular relevance is the finding of Bandura et al.(1987) that persons who report a high level of self-efficacy with regard to pain control (e.g. the belief that one can engage in behavior which will successfully reduce pain) demonstrate greater pain tolerance apparently through the activation of endogenous opioids. As importantly, these authors found that training in cognitive strategies can significantly increase perceived self-efficacy for pain control.

Perhaps of all psychological variables relevant to a discussion of chronic pain none is more clinically compelling than the problem of depression (Romano and Turner, 1985). It is conventional wisdom and beyond dispute that depressed patients reliably report a variety of pain symptoms (Vonknorring, 1975) and that successful treatment of their depression will lead to resolution of their pain (Ward et al., 1979). More frequently depression is one of several behavioral sequelae of chronic pain (Sternbach, 1974). The inextricable link between chronic pain and depression has led some writers to suggest that chronic pain syndromes represent a variant of the spectrum of depressive disorders (Blumer and Heilbronn, 1982). While this view has serious shortcomings (Gupta, 1986; Turk and Salovey, 1984), it does appear that depression and chronic pain share common neurobiological origins (Fields, 1991).

In this regard, the utilization of tricyclic antidepressants (TCA) in the treatment of chronic pain has been a valuable asset to the pain clinician (Monk and Merskey, 1989). Early studies suggested that TCA brought about reductions in pain by virtue of their impact on depressive affect (Turkington, 1980, Ward et al., 1979). Recent evidence has established that the analgesic benefits of TCA are independent of depression. A review of relevant, controlled outcome studies concludes that TCA are an effective pain therapy for a wide array of pain syndromes including post-herpetic neuralgia (Watson et al, 1982), central (thalamic) pain (Leijon and Borie, 1989), diabetic neuropathy (Max et al., 1987), and migraine headaches (Couch and Hassanien, 1976). No data are available for their use in chronic pelvic pain.

Given the multifactorial problems endemic to chronic pain, and the potential contribution of psychological therapies in its management, it is now standard protocol for persistent pain states to be evaluated and treated within a multidisciplinary context (Lorenz, 1981). Pain clinics and programs attempt to address both the medical and psychosocial problems associated with chronic pain, in part by focusing on the suffering and disability aspects of the condition (Fordyce, 1988). By broadening the conceptualization of chronic pain beyond matters of nocioception and tissue damage, this approach has been found to reduce pain and enhance function where circumscribed medical interventions have failed (Aronoff et al., 1985).

ADHESIONS AND PAIN

The etiology of pelvic pain from adhesive disease has been proposed as activation of nociceptors which result from increased tension and traction on the pelvic organs including the ovaries, fallopian tubes, and especially if bowel is involved (Lundberg et al., 1973). The peritoneum is involved in many adhesions and seems to be highly sensitive to nociceptive inputs of stretching and pulling(Bonica, 1990b). Kresch et al. (1984) has proposed that painful adhesions may be qualitatively different from nonpainful adhesions. In his study of 100 patients with chronic pelvic pain, those with pain and adhesions (38%) were felt to have adhesions restricting organ motion and expansibility when compared to control patients without pain but with adhesions (12%). On the other hand, Rapkin (1986) found no significant difference in the density or location of adhesions when comparing women with adhesions and pain to women with infertility, adhesions, and no pain . Stout et al. (1991) also found no correlation between the amount of pathology and self-reported pain in patients with adhesions or endometriosis.

In order to prove a cause and effect relationship between adhesions and pain, it is necessary to show that a significant number of patients with adhesions have pelvic pain. It would also be helpful to show that successful lysis of adhesions results in pain relief. Laparoscopy is the standard diagnostic technique for adhesions, and patients do not undergo laparoscopy without indications such as pain, infertility, or a desire for sterilization. For this reason it is difficult to determine the incidence of pelvic adhesions in the general population and the rate at which patients with adhesions have pelvic pain.

Pelvic adhesions are known to result from tissue damage caused by pelvic surgery, pelvic infection, and endometriosis (Stovall et al., 1989). Yet not all patients with adhesions are noted to have historical predictors of adhesions. History and physical examination have both been found to be poor predictors of pelvic adhesions (Stovall et al., 1989). In a series of laparoscopies performed for diagnosis of pelvic pain, the incidence of patients with adhesions varies between 6 and 55 percent (Steege et al., 1991). In several studies including "control" laparoscopies (i.e., laparoscopies for sterilization or infertility) the incidence of patients with adhesions varies between 14 and 39 percent (Steege et al., 1991). Unfortunately, these "control" patients were not all questioned regarding pain symptoms.

Another way to demonstrate a causative relationship between pelvic adhesions and pelvic pain would be to show that successful lysis of adhesions results in pain relief. Unfortunately, these data are inconclusive for many reasons but most importantly due to the lack of consistency in the measurement of pain and pain relief, and the well recognized consequence of adhesions reformation after adhesiolysis (Diamond and Hershlag, 1990). Stovall and Ling (1991) reported a 48% incidence of adhesions in women with chronic pelvic pain which was not significantly different from a 33.6% incidence of adhesions in their overall population. Adhesiolysis was undertaken in 43 of 229 patients found to have adhesions. Twenty eight (65.1%) were noted to have complete or partial pain relief after 6 months. Nine (20.9%) reported no change in their pain and five (11.6%) reported their pain to be worse . They did not describe the selection criteria for adhesiolysis, the nature of the adhesions present, or what criteria were used to determine response to surgery. They also did not compare their results to changes in pain for those patients who did not undergo adhesiolysis.

Chan and Wood (1985) in Australia obtained similar results. One hundred patients underwent laparotomy with adhesiolysis for infertility, tubal disease, or pelvic pain. The stated operative goal was restoration of normal anatomy. Of 43 women reporting chronic abdominal pain (excluding dysmenorrhea) preoperatively, 28 (65.1%) were either cured or improved based on questionnaire follow-up a minimum of 6 months postoperatively. Nine (20.9%) were unchanged, and 5 (11.6%) were worse. Again, the nature and quantity of the adhesions lysed were not described.

Mecke et al. (1988) in Germany reported only 38% of 52 patients with chronic pelvic pain and adhesions were pain free six months after complete laparoscopic adhesiolysis. An additional 15% noted some reduction in their pain.

In looking at patients following adhesiolysis for chronic pelvic pain, Steege and Stout (1991) were able to show 75% improvement in pain for patients who did not fit their criteria for a chronic pain syndrome, that is, did not exhibit vegetative signs of depression or report altered family roles. Those patients suffering chronic pain syndrome were much less likely to benefit from lysis of adhesions (40%) and pain relief had a greater tendency to be only short term. This is consistent with previous findings that evidence for depression prior to surgery will predict increased severity of pain post-operatively (Jamison et al., 1987; Taenzer et al., 1986).

None of the adhesiolysis studies in women with pelvic pain include evaluation of the success of adhesiolysis with second look laparoscopies. Improvement in symptoms has not been correlated with quantitative decreases in adhesions present. Studies which have been done evaluating adhesion recurrence after adhesiolysis show recurrences in 55-100% of patients (Diamond and Hershlag, 1990). In reviewing the success of adhesiolysis in reproductive surgery these authors note that adhesion reformation seems to be independent of the type of initial adhesions (vascular versus filmy) and that the de novo adhesion rate was significant (31%).

In summary, the available data which correlate the presence of adhesions with the presence of pain are difficult to interpret. The incidence of adhesions confirmed on laparoscopy in patients with and without pain is in the same range. There does seem to be a relationship between adhesiolysis and pain relief suggesting that adhesions are related to pelvic pain, but adhesiolysis is clearly not the cure that most patients are seeking.

CONCLUSION

With multiple studies showing variable and only modest rates of significant pain relief following adhesiolysis, it may be best to consider alternative treatment modalities for patients suffering chronic pelvic pain with adhesions. Several studies have been reported evaluating the effectiveness of multidisciplinary clinics in treating all types of chronic pain (Aronoff et al., 1985). By adopting the multidisciplinary approach popular in the treatment of chronic pain syndromes, perhaps more reliable positive results can be obtained for the treatment of chronic pelvic pain. In this regard, Peters et al (1991) randomized chronic pelvic pain patients to either "standard" or "integrative" approaches to evaluation and treatment. The standard approach routinely included diagnostic laparoscopy and only if no pathology was identified were patients considered for psychological evaluation. The integrative approach paid equal attention to possible organic, psychologic, dietary, and environmental causes of pain. At one year follow-up, using recognized measures of pain severity and function, the group receiving the integrated-approach reported significant improvement in general pain experience, disturbance of daily activities, and associated symptoms when compared to the standard-approach group. The authors concluded that the surgical approach to patients with chronic pelvic pain has been overemphasized, and that a biopsychosocial treatment approach could result in fewer surgical interventions and better improvement in patient's quality of daily life. In a related finding, the availability of multidisciplinary services in a pelvic pain clinic has been shown to decrease the incidence of hysterectomy for chronic pain (Reiter et al, 1991).

Kames et al. (1990) studied chronic pelvic pain patients with and without identifiable pathology within a multi-disciplinary chronic pain program. Patients received a variety of somatic and behavioral therapies, including tricyclic antidepressants, trigger point injections, stress management and self-control procedures, cognitive therapy and sex education. Compared to waiting list controls, treated patients reported a significant decrease in levels of pain, depression and anxiety and improvements in psychosocial functioning including return to work.

If the goal of surgical intervention is a pain free state, published studies cannot support continued emphasis on operative intervention as the only means of treatment. If the goal is pain management, then studies must be undertaken where the surgical outcome is measured in terms of factors critical to a patient's quality of life, including mood and functional ability. Surgical outcome must then be compared to treatment outcome obtained in multidisciplinary pain clinics where surgical intervention is seen as only one arm of treatment. Only when these studies are available will the role of adhesiolysis in the treatment of chronic pelvic pain be more clearly understood. The treatment of women with adhesions and chronic pelvic pain will then be able to focus on what will yield the best outcome for the individual patient.

REFERENCES

Aronoff GM (ed.) (1985): "Evaluation and Treatment of Chronic Pain." Baltimore: Urban and Schwarzenberg.

Aronoff GM, Evans WO, Enders PL (1985): A review of follow-up studies of multidisciplinary pain units. In Aronoff GM (ed.): "Evaluation and Treatment of Chronic Pain." Baltimore: Urban and Schwarzenberg, pp 511-22.

Bandura A, O'Leary A, Taylor CB, Gauthier J, Gossard D (1987): Perceived self-efficacy and pain control: Opioid and nonopioid mechanisms. J Pers Soc Psych, 53:563-71.

Beard RW, Pearce S (1989): Gynaecological pain. In Melzack R, Wall PD (eds) "Textbook of Pain." Edinburgh: Churchill Livingstone, pp 466-81.

Blumer D, Heilbronn M (1982): Chronic pain as a variant of depressive disease: the pain-prone disorder. J Ner Ment Dis, 170:381-406.

Bonica JJ (1990a): Biochemistry and modulation of nocioception and pain. In Bonica JJ (ed.) "The Management of Pain". Malverne: Lea & Febiger, pp 95-121.

Bonica JJ (1990b): General considerations of abdominal pain. In Bonica JJ (ed.) "The Management of Pain." Malverne: Lea & Febiger, pp 1146-85.

Chan CLK, Wood C (1985): Pelvic adhesiolysis-the assessment of symptom relief by 100 patients. Aust NZ J Obstet Gynecol 25:295-8.

Cooper JR, Bloom FE, Roth RH (1982): "The Biochemical Basis of Neuropharmacology." New York: Oxford.

Couch JR, Hassanien RS (1976): Migraine and depression: effect of amitriptyline prophylaxis. Trans Am Neuro Assoc 101:1-4.

Descartes R (1664): L'homme; translated by M Foster (1901): Lectures on the history of physiology during the 16th, 17th, and 18th centuries. Cambridge: Cambridge University Press.

Diamond MP, Hershlag A (1990): Adhesion formation / reformation. In diZerega GS, Malinak LR, Diamond MP, Linsky CB (eds) "Treatment of Post Surgical Adhesions." New York: Wiley-Liss, Inc. pp 23-33.

Engel G (1959): "Psychogenic" pain and the pain-prone patient. Am J Med 26:899-918.

Fields HL (1987): "Pain." New York: McGraw-Hill, Inc.

Fields HL (1991): Depression and pain: a neurobiological model. Neuropsychiatry, Neuropsychology and Behavioral Neurology 4: 83-91.

Fields HL (1984): Brainstem mechanisms of pain modulation. In Kruger L and Liebeskind JC (eds): "Advances in Pain Research and Therapy." Vol. 6. New York: Raven Press, pp 242-52.

Fields HL, Basbaum AI (1979): Anatomy and physiology of a descending pain control system. In Bonica JJ, et al.(ed). "Advances in Pain Research." Vol 3. New York: Raven Press, pp 427-40.

Fordyce WE (1988): Pain and suffering: a reappraisal. Am Psych 43:276-83.

Fordyce WE (1976): "Behavioral Methods for Chronic Pain and Illness." St. Louis: C.V. Mosby.

Getto CJ, Sorkness CA, Howell T (1987): Antidepressants and chronic nonmalignant pain: a review. J Pain and Symp Manage 2:9-18.

Gupta MA (1986): Is chronic pain a variant of depressive illness?: a critical review. Can J Psych 31:241-48.

Guzinski GM (1990): Gynecologic pain. In Bonica JJ (ed). "The Management of Pain." Malverne: Lea & Febiger, pp 1344-67.

Heilman KM Valenstein E (1979): "Clinical Neuropsychology." New York: Oxford.

Henker FO (1979): Diagnosis and treatment of nonorganic pelvic pain. South Med J 72:1132-4.

Hillman P, Wall PD (1969): Inhibitory and excitatory factors influencing the receptive fields of lamina 5 spinal cord cells. Exper Brain Res 9:284-306.

Hughes J, Smith TW, Kosterlitz HN, Fothergill LA, Morgan BA, Morris HR (1975): Identification of two related pentapeptides from the brain with potent opiate, agonist activity. Nature 258:577-9.

Jamison RN, Parris WCV, Maxson WS (1987): Psychological factors influencing recovery from outpatient surgery. Behav Res Ther 25:31-7.

Jensen MP, Turner JA, Romano JM, Karoly P (1991): Coping with chronic pain: a critical review of the literature. Pain 47:249-83.

Kames LD, Rapkin AJ, Naliboff BD, Afifi S, Ferrer-Brechner T (1990): Effectiveness of an interdisciplinary pain management program for the treatment of chronic pelvic pain. Pain 41:41-6.

Keefe FJ, Gil KM (1986): Behavioral concepts in the analysis of chronic pain syndromes. J Cons Clin Psych 54:776-83.

Kresch AJ, Seifer DB, Sachs LB, Barrese I (1984): Laparoscopy in 100 women with chronic pelvic pain. Obstet Gynecol 64:672-4.

Leijon G, Bovie J (1989): Central post-stroke pain: a controlled trial of amitriptyline and carbamazepine. Pain: 36: 27-36.

Lorenz KY Ng (ed.) (1981): New approaches to treatment of chronic pain: a review of multidisciplinary pain clinics and pain center. NIDA Research Monograph 3G. Rockville, MD.

Lundberg WI, Wall JE, Mathers JE (1973): Laparoscopy in evaluation of pelvic pain. Obstet Gynecol 42:872-6.

Mahoney MJ (1977): Reflections on the cognitive-learning trend in psychotherapy. Am Psych 32:5-31.

Mason ST (1984): "Catecholamines and Behavior". Cambridge: Cambridge University Press.

Max MB, Culnane M, Schafer SC, Gracely RH, Walther DJ, Smoller B, Dubner R (1987): Amitryptyline relieves diabetic neuropathy pain in patients with normal or depressed mood. Neurology 37: 589-96.

Mecke H, Semm K, Lehmann-Willenbrock E (1988): [Pelviscopic adhesiolysis. Successes in the treatment of chronic abdominal pain caused by adhesions in the lower and middle abdomen. Gertursholfe Frauenheilkd 48:155-9. (published in German).

Melzack R, Wall PD (1983): "The Challenge of Pain." New York: Basic Books, Inc.

Melzack R, Casey KL (1968): Sensory, motivational, and central control determinants of pain: a new conceptual model. In Kenshalo D (ed), "The Skin Senses." Springfield: Thomas pp 423-43.

Melzack R, Wall PD (1965): Pain mechanisms: a new theory. Science 150:971-979.

Monks R, Merskey H (1989). Psychotropic drugs. In Melzack R, Wall PD (eds). "Textbook of Pain." Edinburgh: Churchill Livingstone, pp 702-21.

Nathan PW (1976): The gate-control theory of pain. Brain 99:123-58.

Peters AAW, van Dorst E, Jellis B, van Zuuren E, Hermans J, Trimbos JB (1991): A randomized clinical trial to compare two different approaches in women with chronic pelvic pain. Obstet Gynecol 77:740-4.

Rapkin AJ (1986): Adhesions and pelvic pain: a retrospective study. Obstet Gynecol 68:13-5.

Reiter RC, Gambone JC, Johnson SR (1991): Availability of a multidisciplinary pelvic pain clinic and frequency of hysterectomy for pelvic pain. J Psych Obstet Gynecol 12(suppl):109-16.

Renaer M. (1980): Chronic pelvic pain without obvious pathology in women. Pain, 106:415-63.

Renaer M, Guzinski GM (1978): Pain in gynecologic practice. Pain 5:305-31.

Romano JA, Turner JA (1985): Chronic pain and depression: does the evidence support a relationship? Psych Bull 97: 18-34.

Selzer M, Spencer WA (1969): Convergence of visceral and cutaneous afferent pathways in the lumbar cord. Brain Res 14:331-48.

Steege JF, Stout AL, Somkuti SG (1991): Chronic pelvic pain in women: toward an integrative model. J Psych Obstet Gynecol 12(suppl):3-30.

Steege JF, Stout AL (1991): Resolution of chronic pelvic pain after laparoscopic lysis of adhesions. Am J Obstet Gynecol 165:278-82.

Sternbach RA (1974): "Pain Patients: Traits and Treatment." New York: Academic.

Stout AL, Steege JF, Dodson WC, Hughes CL (1991): Relationship of laparoscopic findings to self report of pelvic pain. Am J Obstet Gynecol 64:73-9.

Stovall TG, Ling FW (1991): Relieving chronic pelvic pain through surgery. Contemp Ob/Gyn 36(April):11-22.

Stovall TG, Elder RF, Ling FW (1989): Predictors of pelvic adhesions. J Repro Med 34:345-8.

Taenzer P, Melzack R, Jeans ME (1986): Influence of psychological factors on postoperative pain, mood and analgesic requirements. Pain 24:331-42.

Trimbos JB, Trimbos-Kemper GCM, Peters AAW, van der Does CD, van Hall EV (1990): Findings in 200 consecutive asymptomatic women having a laparoscopic sterilization. Arch Gynecol Obstet 247:121-4.

Turk D, Meichenbaum D, Genest M (1983): "Cognitive Therapy of Pain." New York: Guilford.

Turk DC, Rudy TE (1986): Assessment of cognitive factors in chronic pain: a worthwhile enterprise? J Cons Clin Psych 54:760-8.

Turk DC, Salovey P (9184): "Chronic pain as a variant of depressive disease": a critical reappraisal. J Nerv Ment Dis 172:398-404.

Turkington RW (1980): Depression masquerading as diabetic neuropathy. J Am Med Assoc 243:1147-50.

Turner JA, Chapman CR (1982a): Psychological interventions for chronic pain: a critical review. I. Relaxation and biofeedback. Pain 12:1-21.

Turner JA, Chapman CR (1982b): Psychological interventions for chronic pain: a critical review: II. Operant conditioning, hypnosis, and cognitive-behavior therapy. Pain 12:23-46.

Vonknorring L (1975): The experience of pain in depressed patients. Neuropsychobiology 1:155-65.

Wall PD (1964): Presynaptic control of impulses at the first central synapse in the cutaneous pathway. Prog Brain Res 12:92-118.

Wall PD (1978): The gate control theory of pain mechanisms: a re-examination and re-statement. Brain 101:1-18.

Walters A (1961): Psychogenic regional pain alias hysterical pain. Brain 84:1-18.

Ward NG, Bloom VL, Friedel RO (1979): The effectiveness of tricyclic antidepressants in the treatment of coexisting pain and depression. Pain 1:331-41.

Watkins LR, Mayer DJ (1982): Organization of endogenous opiate and nonopiate pain control systems. Science 216:1185-92.

Watson CP, Evans RJ, Reed K, Merskey H. Goldsmith L, Warsh J (1982): Amitriptyline versus placebo in postherpetic neuralgia. Neurology 32:671-3.

Woodforde JM, Mersky H (1972): Personality traits of patients with chronic pain. J Psychoso Res 16:167-72.

Gynecologic Surgery and Adhesion Prevention, pages 121–127

PREVENTION OF ADHESIONS IN OVARIAN SURGERY

Ivo Brosens, M.D., Ph.D.
Professor of Obstetrics and Gynaecology
Director of the Center for Surgical Technologies
University Hospital Gasthuisberg
B 3000 Leuven, Belgium

Postoperative ovarian adhesive disease is the most frequent indication for repeat laparotomy in benign gynaecological conditions by causing infertility, pelvic pain, ovarian cysts and dysfunctional bleeding.

The ovarian surface is a portion of the broader peritoneal surface. When this epithelial surface is resting its cells are mesothelial, but when stimuli serve as irritants, these cells become proliferative. In addition stromal proliferation, metaplasia of peritoneal inclusions and smooth muscle formation are associated with the proliferation of the epithelium.

Ovarian surgery is known to be associated with a major risk of adhesion formation. Microsurgery, laser techniques and endoscopic surgery have been proposed to reduce the risk of adhesion formation. Experimental data of de Waart et al (1987) support the view that after laparoscopic electrocoagulation the risk of adhesion formation is lower than after microsurgical resection (Table 1).

Table 1. Presence and extent of adhesions following microsurgical wedge resection and laparoscopic electrocoagulation of the ovary.

	Microsurgery	Laparoscopic electrocoagulation
	Number of ovaries	
Adhesions	12	12
None	1	11
Mild	5	1
Moderate or severe	6	0

from de Waart et al., 1987

It is therefore important that surgical techniques are used which produce minimal trauma and are associated with reduced risk of adhesion formation.

1. SURGICAL EXPLORATION

Ovarian cysts are frequently an indication for surgical exploration. Women with an apparently benign ovarian cyst can be explored after full work-up by ovarian cystoscopy. According to Bruhat (1991) the risk of laparoscopic error between benign and malignant disease in this group of patients is low (Table 2).

Table 2. Correlation between laparoscopic diagnosis and histologic diagnosis

Laparoscopic diagnosis	N	Histological diagnosis Functional	Organic benign	Border-line	Malignant
Functional	76	67	9	0	0
Organic benign	309	10	299	0	0
Suspect	12	0	8	4	0
Malignant	5	0	0	1	4
Total	402	77	316	5	4

after M. Bruhat, 1989

Brosens and Puttemans (1989) described a double optic technique for ovarioscopy. After aspiration and flushing the content of the cyst, the cystoscopy is performed by a second endoscope consisting of a 5 mm sheath and an optic. The sheath is connected with a saline drip and allows introduction of a biopsy forceps. The sheath with the optic is introduced through a small opening in the ovarian capsule. A saline drip is used to distend the cyst and to allow full inspection of the wall and selection of the sites for biopsies.

The technique has been applied in patients with haemorrhagic ovarian cysts and proved to be useful in two aspects. First, for the in situ differential diagnosis between an ovarian endometrial cyst and a haematoma of the ovary such as a haemorrhagic corpus luteum and second, to examine the type of ovarian endometrioma. Two types or stages of ovarian endometrioma can be distinguished.

The first type is an endometrioma without a fibrotic capsule. The wall of the endometrioma is largely a white, non vascularized surface and can be identified as the inverted ovarian cortex (Fig 1). Mucosa-like endometrial implants, irregular vascularization and adhesions are seen on the wall.

The second type is an endometrioma with a fibrotic capsule. Much of the fibrotic capsule appears as a dark, non-vascularized lining sometimes with a mozaic-like pattern and irregularly distributed vascularized areas. Congested vessels seem to occur more frequently close to the hilus of the ovary.

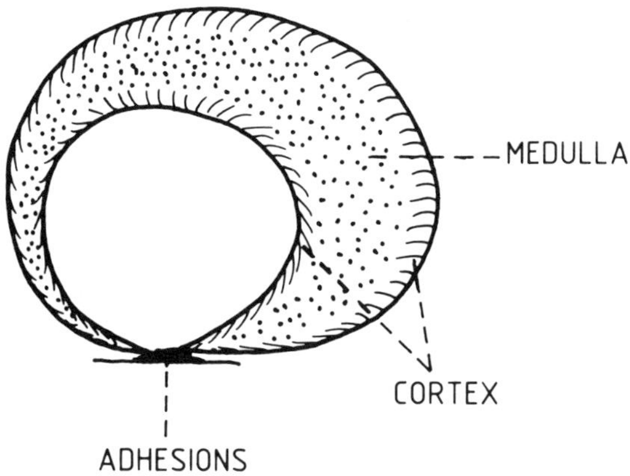

Fig 1 The development of a large ovarian endometrioma by adhesion formation, inversion of the ovarian capsule and distension of the wall. Endometrial foci are implanted on the inverted ovarian cortex.

2. EXCISION OR COAGULATION ?

Excision is indicated for benign neoplastic structures. Two techniques of resection can be used (Bruhat, 1989):
1. After puncture a circular incision is made at the dome of the cyst with scissors and the wall of the cyst is individualized. The plane of cleavage is found by traction on the cyst using a grasping forceps. It is sometimes easier to push the ovarian tissue down than pulling on the cyst. Hemostasis is performed when the vessels at the hilus of the cyst are identified.
2. The ovarian capsule is incised at the dome of the ovarian cyst before puncture and aspiration. The plane of cleavage is made by an atraumatic forceps and/or scissors. The puncture is performed after the wall of the cyst has been dissociated. This technique is used when the nature of the cyst is known before the puncture and is particularly applicable for para-ovarian cyst.

The management of the ovarian endometrioma is a subject of debate. There is a general agreement that endometrioma's of 3 cm or smaller can be treated by adhesiolysis and coagulation. Larger endometrioma's are frequently resected. The dissection can be difficult particularly in the region of the hilus of the ovary.

A three step technique has been proposed by Donnez (1990) (Table 3). We use in specific cases a modified three step technique (Fig 2).

Table 3. Three-step technique of laparoscopic treatment of large ovarian endometrial cyst (J. Donnez 1990)

1. Adhesiolysis, vaporization of peritoneal implants of small (< 3 cm) endometriomas and washing (with saline solution) ovarian cysts > 3 cm of diameter.
2. Hormonal therapy for 3 months (GnRH agonist).
3. Second-look laparoscopy for laser vaporization of residual ovarian cysts.

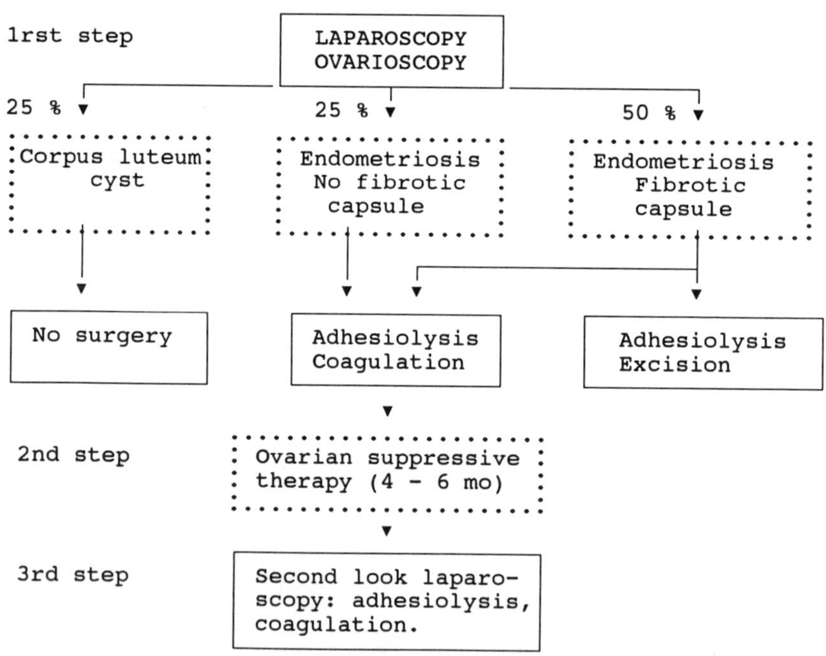

Fig 2 Laparoscopic treatment of the large hemorrhagic cyst of the ovary

The first step involves adhesiolysis, ovarioscopy and coagulation by endo-ovarian argon-laser. The argon laser is color-dependent which means that it is preferentially absorbed by pigments of its complementary color and not by water and therefore can be used inside the ovarian cyst to coagulate the implants and vessels when saline is used to distend the cyst. If the cyst does not remain intact at adhesiolysis the coagulation is performed as described by Donnez (1990).

The second step is a period of ovarian suppressive therapy using a progestogen or a GnRH agonist during a 4 to 6 month period to obtain maximal regression of the cyst.

The third step is a second laparoscopy. At this time the ovarian cyst is usually reduced to a few centimeters or has disappeared and the remaining adhesions and implants of endometriosis are removed. The advantages of this technique is the minimalization of the surgical trauma to the ovarian capsule.

3. CLOSURE OR NOT-CLOSURE ?

Microsurgery.

A microsurgical technique for repair of the ovary as described by Boeckx et al (1980) was applied in 92 patients with ovarian endometriosis (moderate: 50, severe: 38 and extensive: 4). The technique includes meticulous hemostasis, separate 5-0 prolene stitches to reconstruct a normal ovarian shape and a continuing 8-0 nylon suture unless abnormal tension is present. In this instance, interrupted 6-0 stitches are placed in an inverted manner, so that the knot falls inside the ovary. Special care is taken to invert the cut edge of the incision so that only smooth ovarian surfaces are opposed. The follow-up of 60 percent of these patients for 4 years or longer showed ovarian adhesive disease in seven (pelvic pain or dyspareunia in three and a functional cyst in four) and a recurrent endometrial cyst in three patients (Brosens et al, 1988).

Operative laparoscopy

In a prospectively randomized study Nezhat et al (1991) have shown that after resection of the ovarian cyst significantly less adhesions occurred when the ovarian cortex was approximated by simply overlapping the cortex than by suturing the cortex using 4-0 PDS (Table 4).

In the rabbit model it was recently shown by Himebaugh et al. (1991) that adhesion formation after wedge resection is due to a combination of exposed suture material and trauma during repair and that adhesion formation can be mi-

Table 4. Distribution of adnexal adhesions following removal of ovarian cysts

	None	Filmy	Dense
No suture used	12	22	3
Suture used (4-0 PDS)	5	6	20

Nezhat et al., 1991

nimized by closing the ovary with less reactive material such as 6-0 monofilament PDS or by leaving the ovary open.

4. THE NON-OPERATED OVARY

Ovarian adhesions can be caused by removal of the surface epithelium following injury (Gillett et al, 1991). Therefore ovarian handling during ovarian surgery may be implicated in the pathogenesis of adhesion formation. During the training period in tubal microsurgery adhesions also occur on the non-operated side (Boeckx, 1982). It may therefore be important to examine the use of preventive measures of adhesion formation not only on the the operated but also on the non-operated ovary in the pelvic surgery.

CONCLUSION

Whatever surgical technique is used in ovarian surgery, adhesions will occur in a number of cases.

Primary prevention is therefore necessary and is based on avoiding unnecessary ovarian surgery and applying explorative techniques with minimal trauma to the ovary.

In conservative ovarian surgery attention should be paid to the atraumatic manipulation of the ovary as adhesions may form on the non-operated ovary. The appropriate surgical technique should be used and depends on the peroperative diagnosis which can be improved by cystoscopy. There is no necessity for suturing the ovarian capsule if the edges can be approximated. For closing the capsule 6-0 or 8-0 monofilament suture material is recommended.

Preventive measures of adhesion formation should be applied not only to the operated but also to the non-operated ovary.

REFERENCES

Boeckx W, (1982): Reconstructive microsurgery of the rabbit oviduct. Academic thesis, K.U.Leuven.

Boeckx W, Gordts S, Brosens I, (1980) Ovarian microsurgery, in Microsurgery in Female Infertility, P.G. Crosignani and B.L. Rubin (eds), Academic Press, pp 59-76.

Brosens I, Boeckx W, Page G, (1988): Microsurgery of ovarian endometriosis. Human Reproduction 3: 365-366.

Brosens IA, Puttemans PJ, (1989): Double-optic laparoscopy. Salpingoscopy, ovarian cystoscopy and endo-ovarian surgery with the argon laser, Baillière's Clinical Obstetrics and Gynaecology, 3, 595 - 608.

Bruhat M, (1989): Coelioscopie Opératoire, Medsi/McGraw-Hill, pp 187-204

de Waart M, Boeckx W, Brosens I, (1987): Pelvic adhesions following microsurgical wedge resection compared to laparoscopic electrocoagulation of the rabbit ovaries. Infertility 10: 33-39.

Donnez J, Nisolle M, Clerckx F, Gillerot S, Bourgonjon D, Wayembergh M, Casanas-Roux F (1990). The ovarian endometrial cyst: the combined (hormonal and surgical) therapy, in LHRH Analogues in Gynaecology, I. Brosens, H.S. Jacobs, B. Runnebaum (eds), Parthenon Publishing, pp 165-175.

Gillet WR, James C, Jetha N, McComb P, (1991): Removal of ovarian surface epithelium from the rabbit ovary. A cause of ovarian adhesions following injury. Fertil. Steril. S47.

Himebaugh KS, Hurd WW, Cofer KF, Gauvin JM, (1991): The etiology of closure-related adhesion formation after wedge resection of the rabbit ovary. Fertil. Steril. S47.

Nezhat C, Nezhat F, (1991): Postoperative adhesion formation after ovarian cystectomy with and without ovarian reconstruction. Fertil. Steril. S47.

Gynecologic Surgery and Adhesion Prevention, pages 129–138

LAPAROSCOPIC OVARIAN DRILLING IN WOMEN WITH POLYCYSTIC OVARIAN SYNDROME

Ellen Mary Greenblatt
Robert F. Casper
Department of Obstetrics and Gynecology
University of Toronto
Toronto, Ontario, M5G 2C4, Canada

INTRODUCTION

In 1935, Stein and Leventhal (1) first described the association of enlarged polycystic ovaries with the clinical features of amenorrhea, obesity and hirsutism. Since then, the polycystic ovarian syndrome (PCOS) has been recognized to be variable in its clinical and biochemical presentation. Despite the variability of presentation, chronic anovulation with evidence of androgen excess remains the hallmark of this syndrome.

A self-perpetuating cycle of biochemical abnormalities has been described in polycystic ovarian disease (2). The pathophysiology of PCOS has been presented in detail in several recent reviews (3,4) and will not be discussed in detail in this paper. The focus of this paper will be on ovulation induction for infertility associated with PCOS. In particular, recent laparoscopic surgical techniques in cases resistant to conventional medical management shall be described. Emphasis will be placed on the description of these techniques, discussing mechanisms of action, success rates, as well as potential risks and complications, particularly related to adhesion formation. Emphasis will be on practical application of these techniques as well as methods to minimize complications.

OVULATION INDUCTION IN PCOS

Medical Treatment. Patients with chronic anovulation and polycystic ovaries generally respond to administration of clomiphene citrate for induction of ovulation.

However, even with the use of increasing doses of clomiphene and the addition of human chorionic gonadotropin, 10% to 15% of women remain anovulatory (5,6,7). For these patients, ovulation induction can be difficult. Subsequent therapy commonly involves daily parenteral administration of human menopausal gonadotropins (hMG) or pure human follicle stimulating hormone (FSH). However, both these medications are costly, require extensive monitoring and are associated with a significant risk of multiple pregnancy and ovarian hyperstimulation syndrome (8,9)

As women with hypothalamic amenorrhea respond more predictably to gonadotropin administration than do women with PCOS, clinicians have attempted use of long acting GnRH agonists to convert the steroidal milieu in women with PCOS to one comparable to that seen in women with hypothalamic amenorrhea prior to hMG administration. These attempts have met with varying success(10,11). Although the incidence of premature luteinization seems to be reduced, that of hyperstimulation is unchanged, and severe hyperstimulation does occur.

Encouraged by the results of pulsatile GnRH administration in hypothalamic amenorrhea, attempts to override the abnormal gonadotropin signal in PCOS with exogenously administered pulsatile GnRH, with or without pretreatment with GnRH analogs, have been variable (12,13, 14).

SURGICAL TREATMENT

Ovarian Wedge Resection. Historically, the approach to ovulation induction in clomiphene resistant women with PCOS has been ovarian wedge resection (OWR) (15,16,17). This treatment fell into disfavour for three reasons. Firstly, a laparotomy was required. Secondly,it became apparent that a significant number of women relapse and therefore the effects may be short lived. Finally, and most importantly, formation of post operative adhesions was common, introducing a mechanical cause of infertility. (18) This problem has not been adequately readdressed in light of advancements in microsurgical approach to infertility surgery (19).

Laparoscopic "Ovarian Drilling." Recently, minimally invasive operative-laparoscopic techniques have been described for the treatment of anovulation in patients with polycystic ovarian disease. The majority of these approaches involve the laparoscopic formation of multiple areas of injury to the surface of the ovary and include, laparoscopic ovarian cautery (20,21,22,23), and laparoscopic ovarian laser vaporization using CO_2, argon and KTP or Nd:YAG laser (24,25). Following either of these procedures, the ovary appears to have been 'drilled' at multiple points along its surface and the popular acronym of 'ovarian drilling' has appeared in the literature in association with these two techniques. Clinical results appear promising with a high rate of successful ovulation and conception occurring without the need for intensive patient monitoring.

Technique of Laparoscopic Ovarian Cautery. This procedure, first described by Gjonnaess (20), involves the use of monopolar electrocautery applied through the laparoscope. Briefly, diagnostic laparoscopy is done in the usual fashion. The presence of polycystic ovaries is documented and tubal patency confirmed with methylene blue hydrotubation. Through a suprapubic or lower quadrant puncture, a second trocar is inserted and an atraumatic grasping forceps is used to stabilize the ovary by holding the ovarian ligament. A third puncture is then placed in the right or left lower quadrant and through this trocar sheath is passed a unipolar cautery instrument with a cone-shaped tip or laparoscopic scissors attached to monopolar cautery. Since it is necessary to penetrate the cortex of the ovary, an instrument with a sharp tip is preferable to one with a rounded or dull tip. The ovary must be carefully held away from bowel and other vital structures since sparking and arcing may occur with monopolar cautery. Using a 4mA current, the diathermy instrument is held against the surface of the ovary until it is seen to penetrate the cortex. This is accompanied by a popping sensation and is often associated with a burst of fluid that exits from small subcortical follicles. A minimum of 10 holes, approximately 3-4 mm in diameter and approximately 5 mm deep, is burned at random over the surface of the ovary avoiding the hilum of the ovary in order to prevent disruption of the ovarian blood supply. The same procedure is then repeated in the other ovary. Following ovarian cautery, the ovaries are cooled by dipping them into a pool of irrigation solution consisting of Ringers Lactate containing 1000U heparin per litre. Hemostasis is achieved, if necessary, with additional use of cautery.

Results of Laparoscopic Ovarian Cautery. In the first report of this technique,(20) 62 women with polycystic ovarian disease and anovulation were treated. Ninety-two percent of the patients ovulated following surgery. Of 35 women desiring pregnancy, 69% became pregnant after cautery alone with a total of 80% conceiving after cautery with addition of clomiphene. Subsequent studies (21,22,23) have confirmed that 80 to 90% of patients will ovulate following ovarian cautery for polycystic ovarian syndrome and conception rates in the range of 45-66% usually are seen in 6-12 months follow-up.

Laparoscopic Laser Vaporization. More recently, the CO_2, argon, KTP and Nd:YAG lasers have been successfully utilized for laparoscopic vaporization of the ovaries in polycystic ovarian disease. (24,25) With the CO_2 laser, 10 or more holes, 3-4mm in diameter, are vaporized on the surface of the ovary. Smoke production may obscure the view of the ovaries with the CO_2 laser and needs to be intermittently vented off, ideally with continuous high flow insufflation of intraperitoneal CO_2. In general, hemorrhage is not a problem during ovarian vaporization even though the CO_2 laser is mainly a cutting tool. If bleeding occurs, use of a monopolar or bipolar cautery may be necessary for hemostasis.

With the use of KTP or argon laser system, a third puncture site is required for introduction of the fiber-optic system. However, the deeper tissue penetration and decrease in smoke formation which are elements of these systems may allow for shorter operating time.

With the Nd:YAG laser, the utilization of a fiberoptic delivery system with sapphire tips for focussing the laser beam allows tissue contact through the laparoscope. This system has resulted in a simple method of vaporization of points on the ovarian capsule with enhanced safety compared to the monopolar cautery technique and with minimal smoke production. Hemostasis is achieved since the Nd:YAG wavelength also produces photocoagulation. The Nd:YAG laser has been used to remove a wedge of tissue (26). Bleeding has not been a complication and the defect is left to heal by secondary intention.

Results of laparoscopic ovarian laser vaporization. Following laser vaporization of the ovaries or laser wedge resection in polycystic ovarian disease, approximately 70-80% of patients ovulate spontaneously in the post-operative period (24-26). In general, patients who do not ovulate spontaneously are rendered responsive to clomiphene. With 6 month follow-up, pregnancy rates in the range of 60% have been reported following laser therapy.

Mechanism of action. Although the mechanism of action of laparoscopic ovarian cautery or laser vaporization in inducing ovulation in patients with PCOS remains unknown, it is thought to be similar to the mechanism of action of ovarian wedge resection.

Steroid and gonadotropin levels prior to and following laparoscopic ovarian cautery have been evaluated in an effort to delineate the mechanism of action of this procedure (21,22,27,28,29). Greenblatt and Casper (21) followed daily hormone levels pre-operatively and for ten days postoperatively. They describe a fall in testosterone, androstenedione, and estradiol on post-op day 3-4 and a rise in FSH on day 2. LH levels rose on day one but subsequently fell to a nadir on day 3. These changes did not occur in a control group of normal women undergoing laparoscopy.

It is speculated that the fall in estradiol may be responsible for decreased positive feedback on LH and decreased negative feedback on FSH at the level of the pituitary. The rise in serum FSH levels occurring in the post operative period may result in increased aromatase activity within the follicles. This effect, coupled with a decrease in local androgen concentrations, would convert the intrafollicular environment from being androgen dominant to one that is estrogenic. As high intrafollicular androgens have been shown to be associated with follicular atresia, the conversion of an androgenic microenvironment within the follicle to an estrogenic one may remove an intraovarian block to follicular maturation, allowing follicular recruitment and development to proceed to subsequent ovulation.

Sumioki et al (27) described a similar fall in LH by postoperative day 4 which was due to a decrease in pulse amplitude but not frequency. The typical increased sensitivity of LH to a GnRH bolus seen in PCO women pre-operatively was decreased post-operatively as well. Testosterone (total and free), androstenedione, and estrone fell reaching a nadir on day 3-4 post surgery. Dehydroepiandrosterone-sulfate which is principally made in the adrenal, showed no consistent change.

In general, the hormonal responses are similar to those following wedge resection (30,31) It is not known why the observed endocrine changes occur following ovarian vaporization or cautery. However, it is possible that they are the result of the destruction of androgen producing tissue in the ovary with resultant decreased conversion to peripheral estrogen and decreased intrafollicular androgen environment. Other possibilities include local factors such as inflammation and increased blood flow with resultant increased delivery of gonadotropins which may result in altered follicular activity. A recent study in which serum inhibin concentrations were measured after ovarian cautery for PCO demonstrated an immediate postoperative decline (32).

Benefits of laparoscopic drilling procedures for PCOS. Anovulatory women with PCOS who fail to respond to therapy with clomiphene citrate are faced with the prospect of ovulation induction with gonadotropins. These women are particularly at risk for hyperstimulation and multiple pregnancy with this form of treatment. Furthermore, gonadotropin therapy is expensive and requires extensive time commitment for adequate follicular monitoring. Prior to committing a patient to this treatment, many clinicians will recommend laparoscopy to evaluate tubal patency and to rule out other disease processes that may be contributing to infertility. Laparoscopic ovarian cautery or laser vaporization at the time of diagnostic laparoscopy adds minimal time or morbidity to the procedure and may circumvent the need for gonadotropin therapy.

A recent prospective, study of 85 infertile, clomiphene resistant women with PCOS evaluated pregnancy rates achieved following randomization to one of three treatments arms: Laparoscopic ovarian electrocautery, hMG or FSH (33). Fifty-two percent, 55% and 38% of women in each group, respectively, conceived within 6 months. Furthermore, all pregnancies were singleton in the ovarian cautery group compared with a 20% multiple pregnancy rate in the other two groups. Pregnancy wastage, was 21%, 53% and 40% respectively (not significantly different) (33). In summary, ovarian cautery seems at least as good as more expensive methods which require ongoing treatment and monitoring.

Complications of Laparoscopic Cautery and Laser Vaporization. No serious complications have been reported with laparoscopic ovarian cautery. However, the use of monopolar cautery carries the potential risk of arcing with damage to adjacent organs, especially bowel. The newer laser techniques of ovarian capsule vaporization appear to be effective in inducing ovulation with less chance of bowel injury than monopolar cautery.

Perhaps a more significant complication is the potential of ovarian drilling procedures to cause adhesion formation. Sporadic reevaluation of ovaries post cautery or vaporization (20,24) have not revealed any adhesions and the high conception rate would suggest that post operative adhesions are not a frequent problem. However a preliminary study has addressed this issue (34). Second look laparoscopies were performed 3-4 weeks after laparoscopic ovarian electrocautery or Nd:YAG laser vaporization in 6 women with polycystic ovarian disease. All 6 laparoscopies revealed ovarian adhesions which were extensive in some cases. However, the adhesions were easily separated by blunt dissection and it was suggested that second look laparoscopy may be needed to prevent permanent adhesion formation with this technique.

A larger study was recently published (35). This group performed short-interval second-look laparoscopy and lysis of adhesions where necessary, at 4-6 weeks in a group of 17 clomiphene-resistant women with polycystic ovarian disease undergoing laparoscopic ovarian cautery (n=7) or ovarian vaporization (n=10) using the Nd:YAG laser (non-contact technique). In this study 14/17 women had post operative adhesions, although these were classified as minimal to mild in 12/14. By 6 months, 4/7 and 4/10 women in the cautery and laser groups, respectively, had conceived.

In an attempt to minimize the undesirable development of post-operative adhesions which introduces a mechanical infertility factor, studies are currently underway to evaluate methods to reduce this problem. Several materials to reduce post-operative adhesion formation following major infertility surgery have been evaluated (36,37,38). Results are variable. Recently, INTERCEED (TC7) Absorbable Adhesion Barrier (Ethicon, Inc., Summerville, N.J.), a fabric composed of oxidized, regenerated cellulose has been evaluated in animal models(39,40), and in women undergoing lysis of adhesions for infertility (41). Results appear promising.

At the University of Toronto, Toronto, Ontario, Canada, we are currently involved in a randomized, blinded, prospective study evaluating the possible role of INTERCEED in prevention of adhesions following laparoscopic ovarian cautery in women with clomiphene resistant PCOS. Women undergoing this procedure have INTERCEED placed over the surface of one ovary, selected at random, at the conclusion of the procedure. Four to 6 weeks later, second-look laparoscopy with classification of adhesions according to the American Fertility Society (42) and lysis of adhesions is performed by a second surgeon unaware of which ovary was treated. Preliminary data comparing the control and Interceed side is limited due to the difficulty in applying Interceed to (43), and assuring oneself that the material remains on, the surface of the ovary. New instruments and methods are currently being investigated to eliminate this problem. However, preliminary data on 5 patients has demonstrated significant adhesion formation, bilaterally, severe in some cases. Until this technique has been further evaluated, laparoscopic ovarian cautery must be considered investigational, and associated with the risk of significant post-operative adhesion formation.

Finally, as with wedge resection, the effects of ovarian drilling procedures may not be permanent (20,22). Thus, this procedure should be reserved for women who are actively trying to conceive.

CONCLUSION

Since the description of polycystic ovarian syndrome by Stein and Leventhal in 1935, advances in our understanding of the pathophysiology and treatment of the problems associated with this syndrome have occurred. Investigators are recognizing the variability in presentation of PCOS. Infertility secondary to anovulation is still the most common reason for a women with PCOS to seek medical treatment. The spectrum of therapeutic approaches for ovulation induction in these women is possibly swinging back to the use of surgical modalities, including laparoscopic ovarian cautery or laser vaporization in an attempt to normalize the follicular environment within polycystic ovaries and allow normal follicular development and ovulation. Future controlled trials aimed at understanding the mode of action of these procedures and reducing post-operative adhesion formation are required before they can be considered part of the routine management of anovulation in PCOS.

REFERENCES

1. Stein IF, Leventhal ML. Amenorrhea associated with bilateral polycystic ovaries. Am J Obstet Gynecol 1935; 29:181.

2. Yen SSC. The polycystic ovary syndrome. Clin Endocrinol 1980;12:177.

3. Shelley DR, Dunaif A. Polycystic ovary syndrome. Comprehensive Therapy 1990;16(11): 26.

4. Barnes R, Rosenfield RL. The polycystic ovary syndrome: Pathogenesis and treatment. Ann Int Med 1989; 110:386.

5. Franks S, Adams J, Mason H, et al. Ovulatory disorders in women with polycystic ovary syndrome. Clin Obstet Gynecol 1985;12:605.

6 Raj SG, Thompson IE, Berger MJ, Taymor ML. Clinical aspects of the polycystic ovary syndrome. Obstet Gynecol 1977:49:552.

7. Gorlitsky GA, Kase NG, Speroff L. Ovulation and pregnancy rates with clomiphene citrate. Obstet Gynecol 1978; 51:265.

8 Wang CF, Gemzell C. The use of human gonadotropins for the induction of ovulation in women with polycystic ovarian disease. Fertil Steril 1980; 33:479.

9 Check JH, Wu CH, Gocial B, et al. Severe ovarian hyperstimulation syndrome from treatment with urinary follicle-stimulating hormone: two cases. Fertil Steril 1985;43:317.

10. Dodson WC, Hughes CL, Whitesides DB, et al. The effect of leuprolide acetate on ovulation induction with human menopausal gonadotropins in polycystic ovary syndrome. J Clin Endocrinol Metab 1987;65:95.

11. Fleming R, Haxton MJ, Hamilton MP, et al. Successful treatment of infertile women with oligomenorrhoea using combination of an LHRH agonist and exogenous gonadotrophins. Br J Obstet Gynaecol 1985; 92:369-373.

12. Bennink HJTC, Weber HW, Alsbach HJ, et al.. Induction of ovulation by pulsatile intravenous administration of GnRH in polycystic ovarian disease. Fertil Steril 1984;41:34s.

13. Burger CW, Korsen TJM, Hompes PGA, et al. Ovulation induction with pulsatile luteinizing releasing hormone in women with clomiphene citrate-resistant polycystic ovary-like disease: clinical results. Fertil Steril 1986;46:1045.

14. Filicori M, Campaniello E, Michelacci L, et al. Gonadotropin-releasing hormone (GnRH) analog suppression renders polycystic ovarian disease patients more susceptible to ovulation induction with pulsatile GnRH. J Clin Endocrinol Metab 1988;66:327.

15. Goldzieher JW, Green JA. The polycystic ovary: Clinical and histological features. J Clin Endocrinol Metab 1962;22:325.

16. Stein I.F., Leventhal M.L. Duration of fertility following ovarian wedge resection--Stein-Leventhal Syndrome.Obstet Gynecol Surv 1965;20:124.

17. Adashi E.Y., Rock J.A., Guzich D, et al. Fertility following bilateral ovarian wedge resection : A critical analysis of 90 consecutive cases of polycystic ovary syndrome. Fertil Steril;1981:36:320.

18. Buttram V, Vaquero C. Post-ovarian wedge resection adhesive disease. Fertil Steril 1975; 26:874.

19. Eddy CA, Asch RH, Balmaceda JP. Pelvic adhesions following microsurgical and macrosurcical wedge resection of the ovaries. Fertil Steril 1980;33:557.

20. Gjonnaess H. Polycystic ovarian syndrome treated by ovarian electrocautery through the laparoscope. Fertil Steril 1984;41:20.

21. Greenblatt E, Casper RF. Endocrine changes after laparoscopic ovarian cautery in polycystic ovarian syndrome. Am J Obstet Gynecol 1987; 156:279-285.

22. Armar N A , McGarrigle HHG, Honour J,et al. Laparoscopic ovarian diathermy in the management of anovulatory infertility in women with polycystic ovaries. Endocrine changes and clinical outcome. Fertil Steril 1990;53:45.

23. van der Weiden RM, Alberda AT. Laparoscopic ovarian electrocautery in patients with polycystic ovarian disease resistant. Surg Endosc 1987;1:217

24. Daniell JF, Miller W. Polycystic ovaries treated by laparoscopic laser vaporization. Fertil Steril 1989;51:232.

25. Huber J, Hosmann J, Spona J. Polycystic ovarian syndrome treated by laser through the laparoscope. Lancet 1988;2:215.

26. Kojima E, Yanagibori A, Otaka K,et al. Ovarian wedge resection with contact Nd:YAG laser irradiation used laparoscopically. J Reprod Med 1989;34:444.

27. Sumioki H, Utsunomyiya T, Matsuoka K, Korenaga M, Kadota, T. The effect of laparoscopic multiple punch resection of the ovary on hypothalamo-pituitary axis in polycystic ovary syndrome. Fertil Steril 1988; 50:567-572.

28.Aakvaag A, Gjonnaess H. Hormonal response to electrocautery of the ovary in patients with polycystic ovarian disease. Br J Obstet Gynaecol 1985;92:1258

29.Gjonnaess H, Norman N. Endocrine effects of ovarian electrocautery in patients with polycystic ovarian disease. Brit. J Obstet Gynaecol 1987;94:779

30. Judd HL, Riggs LA, Anderson DC, et al. The effects of ovarian wedge resection on circulating gonadotropin and ovarian steroid levels in patients with polycystic ovary syndrome. J Clin Endocrinol Metab 1976;43:346.

31. Katz M, Carr PJ, Cohen BM,et al. Hormonal effects of wedge resection in polycystic ovaries. Obstet Gynecol 1978;51:437.

32. Kovacs G, Buckler H, Bangah, M,et al. Treatment of anovulation due to polycystic ovarian syndrome by laparoscopic ovarian electrocautery. Brit J Obstet Gynaec 1991;98:30.

33. Abdel Gadir A, Mowafi R.S., Anlaser H.M.I. et al. Ovarian electrocautery versus human menopausal donadotrphins and pure follicle stimulating hormone therapy in the treatment of patients with polycystic ovarian disease. Clin Endocrinol. 1990;33:585.

34. Lyles R, Goldzieher JW, Betts JW, et al. Early second look laparoscopy after the treatment of polycystic ovarian disease with laparoscopic ovarian electrocautery and/or ND:YAG laser photocoagulation. (Abstract 0-061) Presented at the 45th Annual Meeting of The American Fertility Society, San Francisco, California, November 13-16,1989. Program Supplement, pS26.

35. Gurgan T, Kisnisci H, Yarali H, et al. Evaluation of adhesion formation after laparoscopic treatment of polycystic ovarian disease. Fertil Steril 1991;56:1176.

36. Holtz G. Prevention of postoperative adhesions. 1980;J. Reprod Med; 24:141.

37. Diamond MP, Danniell JF, Feste J, et al. Adhesion reformation and de novo adhesion formation after reproductive pelvic surgery. Fertil Steril 1987;47:864.

38. Diamond MP, DeCherney AH, Linsky CB et al. Assessment of carboxymethylcellulose and 32% Dextran 70 for prevention of adhesions in a rabbit uterine horn model. Int J Fertil 1988;33:278.

39. Diamond MP, Linsky CB, Cunningham TJ et al. A model for sidewall adhesions in the rabbit; reduction by an absorbable barrier. Microsurgery 1987;8:197

40. Linsky CB Diamond MP, Cunningham TJ et al. Adhesion reduction in the uterine horn model using an absorbable barrier, TC7. J Reprod Med 1987;32:17.

41. INTERCEED (TC7) Adhesion Barrier Study Group: Prevention of postsurgical adhesions by INTERCEED (TC7), an absorbable adhesion barrier: A prospective, randomized multicenter clinical study. Fertil Steril 1989;51:933.

42. The American Fertility Society: The American Fertility classification of adnexal adhesions, distal tubal occlusion secondary to tubal ligation, tubal pregnancies, Mullerian anomalies, and intrauterine adhesions. Fertil Steril 1988;49:944

43. Azziz R, Murphy AA, Rosenberg SM, et al. Use of an oxidized, regenerated cellulose absorbable adhesion barrier at laparoscopy. J Reprod Med 1991;36:479.

Gynecologic Surgery and Adhesion Prevention, pages 139–147

TREATMENT OF ECTOPICS AND SUBSEQUENT ADHESION FORMATION

Per Lundorff
Department of Obstetrics and Gynecology
Sahlgrenska Hospital
Gothenburg, Sweden

Infertility after ectopic pregnancy (EP) is well documented (Sherman, et al., 1982, Tuomivaara and Kauppila, 1988, Thorburn, et al., 1988). To a certain extent the subsequent infertility may be the result of the operative trauma to the fallopian tubes and formation of new pelvic adhesions. Interest has therefore been focused on more conservative treatments of EP, including laparoscopic techniques (Bruhat, et al., 1980).

Periadnexal adhesion formation is an important factor in infertility after pelvic surgery, and evaluation of the etiology and prevention of adhesion formation have been the major goal for many investigations (Myhre-Jensen, et al., 1969, Levinson and Swolin, 1980). Normal peritoneum has an inherent fibrinolytic activity (Myhre-Jensen, et al., 1969, Porter, et al., 1969). Peritoneal defects, if left open and vascularized, heal rapidly by fibroblast differentiation into a smooth new serosa (Ellis, 1980). Experimental studies in the rat show that local ischemia hampers the ability of the peritoneum to perform spontaneous fibrinolysis (Raftery, 1981). The inherent response to the presence of ischaemic peritoneal tissue is adhesion formation, which acts as vascular grafts (Ellis, 1980).

To avoid tissue ischemia and adhesion formation in the operation field, Levinson and Swolin (1980) advocated nontraumatic techniques with bloodless entry into the abdominal cavity by use of electrosurgery, peritoneal lavage and complete excision of diseased tissue. Peritoneal lavage with different concentrations of corticosteroids, non steroidal anti-inflammatory agents and high molecular weight solutions for adhesion prophylaxis has been shown to be valuable (Swolin, 1967, Rosenburg and Board, 1983).

Efforts also are directed toward early recognition of EP and thereby earlier surgical intervention with reduced damage to the pelvic organs. The value of postoperative laparoscopy at intervals from 8 days to 8 weeks or longer after conventional microsurgery for infertility has been assessed by several author (Ray and Hulka, 1982, DeCherney and Mezer, 1984, Trimbos-Kemper, et al., 1985, Jansen, 1988). An early second-look laparoscopy makes adhesiolysis easier and formation of thick and vascular adhesions is reduced.

The presence of adhesions is also suggested to be of great importance for subsequent fertility (Caspi, et al., 1979) and adhesiolysis among infertility patients is recommended (Bronson and Wallach, 1977, Tulandi, et al., 1990). Efforts have consequently been concentrated on minimizing the formation of adhesions, e.g., by using laparoscopic treatment (Pouly, et al., 1986).

At the department of Obstetrics and Gynecology, Sahlgrenska Hospital, Gothenburg, Sweden, we wanted to analyze whether a classification system could be applied to assess the pelvic status in connection with EP surgery. Our intention was to analyze whether various surgical procedures differ in respect of the pelvic status at the time of second-look laparoscopy. For this purpose a modification of a preoperative classification scheme was used. This classification was based on a scoring system according to tubal damage and adhesions intended for prediction of the intrauterine and EP rates after distal microsurgery (Mage, et al., 1986).

MATERIAL AND METHODS

In a retrospective study (Lundorff, et al., 1990), 102 women with a strong desire for pregnancy underwent second-look laparoscopy about 6 to 10 weeks after primary surgery. The study was based on records and peroperative illustrations from these 102 women, and we used the scoring system (Mage, et al., 1986), with minor modifications, to classify pelvic findings during and after EP surgery, with respect to both tubal damage and adhesions. Our analysis thus comprises: (1) a score for the contralateral tube and (2) a score for the adhesions of both sides. Furthermore, peroperative intervention such as lysis of adhesions was noted.

At the time of second-look laparoscopy, the same classification system was used and new scores were calculated, thus making it possible to determine a "score change". Tubal patency for both tubes was registered, interventions such as lysis of adhesions were noted, and the prognosis for future fertility was evaluated for all patients. The patients were separated into different groups according to the method of surgery in order to determine whether any method was superior with respect to patency of the oviducts or prevention of adhesions and tubal damage.

Of all patients 42% had a salpingotomy performed by laparotomy, 21% underwent expressio ovi, 21% had a salpingotomy performed by laparoscopy, 12% had a tubal resection, and 3% had a salpingectomy performed. Two patients were evacuated from a Douglas pouch hematoma. Furthermore, two women, who previously had a salpingectomy performed on the contralateral tube, were sterilized in connection with this EP surgery intended for future IVF treatment. Laparoscopic treatment, when used, was performed by electrocautery, linear salpingotomy and suction-irrigation. No women underwent a laparoscopic salpingectomy.

At the time of EP surgery, lysis of adhesions was performed in 23 patients (22.5%). Of these 23 women, 7 presented with less adhesions at the second-look laparoscopy on the affected side. Nine patients were improved on the contralateral side and 5 patients were improved on both sides.

At the second-look laparoscopy, lysis was performed in 42 patients (41.2%). In 4 patients advanced adhesions hampered lysis via the laparoscope. In two patients, sterilization was performed with the intention of future IVF treatment.

Classification of the Pelvic Status at the Second-look Laparoscopy

On both sides, tubal patency was present in about 70% of all cases.

An equal tubal score was present in 80 patients (87%), nine patients (10%) were impaired and three patients (3%) were improved. Lysis of adhesions had been performed at the first surgical intervention in all three cases, where improvement was noted.

Adhesions On the affected side impairment of the adhesions between the two surgical procedures was noted in 40 patients (39%). Forty-eight patients (47%) had an unchanged status whereas 14 patients (14%) had an improved status. Seven of the latter women underwent lysis of adhesions during the first surgical intervention.

On the contralateral side, 23 patients (22%) had an impairment of the adhesions, 68 patients (67%) were unchanged and 11 patients (11%) presented an improvement, i.e. a lower score. Nine of the latter patients underwent lysis of adhesions during the first operation.

CLASSIFICATION FOR FUTURE FERTILITY

In 67 cases, at least one tube was classified as normal and the anatomical condition of the pelvis was considered satisfactory. These patients were not subjected to further surgical intervention during the first year of observation. In 13 cases the probability of future pregnancy was considered extremely low because of adhesions and/or tubal damage. These patients were therefore offered microsurgery. More advanced damage to the tubes or severe adhesions were found in 12 women and microsurgery was considered meaningless, as it was in two patients sterilized at EP surgery. These 14 women were offered IVF treatment or recommended adoption. Gamete intrafallopian transfer (GIFT) was offered in one case. The remaining 7 patients were recommended hysterosalpingography for further evaluation of the anatomical conditions.

Comparison Between Surgical Methods

There was no correlation between surgical methods and tubal patency.

Tubal and Adhesion Score

No surgical procedure was found to be correlated to improvement or impairment of adhesions or tubal score. Thus, a laparoscopic treatment did not imply less adhesions at second-look laparoscopy compared with conventional laparotomy. Subjective evaluation of the degree of adhesions by different surgeons may also have contributed to a certain bias. In spite of this, we found it most valuable to study possible benefits of a second-look laparoscopy in routine clinical practice and to investigate whether there were any special conditions leading to an impairment of the pelvic status after EP surgery.

Based on results from our study, it is thus not possible to determine which patients will develop an impairment of adhesions after EP surgery. As we found that almost every second woman in our material presented an impairment of adhesions, we suggest that all patients with a desire for pregnancy should be offered a second-look laparoscopy. Our results further indicate that patency is not seen more frequently after laparoscopic treatment than after conservative treatment by laparotomy. Neither could we demonstrate less frequent adhesions after laparoscopic treatment than after conservative treatment by laparotomy. However, as this study is not a randomized prospective trial, no conclusions can be drawn in that respect. Surprisingly, we found that a large proportion of the patients had undergone lysis of adhesions at the EP operation. This is generally not recommended (Winston and Margara, 1984). Nevertheless, we observed that half of the patients subjected to lysis of adhesions at the time of EP surgery presented an improved status at the time of the second-look laparoscopy. Nearly 40% of all the patients presented an impairment of the pelvic status at the second-look laparoscopy and as many were treated by lysis of adhesions. To what extent such adhesiolysis will contribute to a better fertility prognosis is not possible to evaluate on the basis of this study.

RANDOMIZED TRIAL

A randomized trial was initiated to study the adhesion formation (Lundorff, et al., 1991a) and the subsequent fertility prospects (Lundorff, 1991c) in women with EP treated either by laparotomy or laparoscopy.

Design

105 women with tubal pregnancies fulfilling the entry criteria (see below), were stratified on the basis of age and risk determinants (Thorburn, et al., 1986) (previous EP, previous abdominal surgery, history of infertility or intrauterine device (IUD) in situ), to establish comparable groups for future fertility evaluation and randomized in a prospective trial to either surgery by laparoscopy (n=48) or laparotomy (n=57) by sealed envelopes (Lundorff, et al., 1991b). All operations were performed under general anesthesia with endotracheal intubation. For the laparoscopic surgery, an 8 to 10 mm laparoscope was used, introduced through the umbilicus. Two

additional 5 mm trocars were inserted suprapubic in the right and left side of the lower pelvis for introduction of a grasping forceps, a diathermy knife and intermittently, a suction - irrigation unit (Aquapurator, Wisap, Sauerlach, Germany). A diluted solution of vasopressin, 5 IU in 10 mL of saline was injected into the mesosalpinx for hemostasis via a 0.8 mm. syringe. The tube was opened with a fine diathermy knife over the implantation site with a longitudinal incision (10 to 15 mm), and the pregnancy products were removed either with the Aquapurator or with 10 mm spoon forceps. In case of laparotomy, vasopressin injection and a salpingotomy with a similar diathermy knife was performed and the pregnancy products squeezed through the opening. All surgical interventions were performed by one of the authors with the aim of performing a linear salpingotomy regardless of the operative approach. An atraumatic, gentle technique was always used. Irrespective of the operative approach, the affected tube was left open for secondary healing. Entry criteria were: (1) diameter of the tubal gestation < 4 cm, (2) ampullary gestation accessible for laparoscopic approach, (3) a trained laparoscopist on duty, and (4) hemodynamic stability. If the preoperative human chorionic gonadotropin level was known, cases with titres above 10,000 IU/L were excluded. A gross anatomy evaluation of the periadnexal and tubal status was undertaken during surgery.

A second-look laparoscopy (Lundorff, et al., 1991a) was performed in mean 12 weeks (range 1 to 29 weeks) after primary surgery in 73 cases with a desire for pregnancy (laparoscopy N=31; laparotomy N=42).

Thirty-two patients had no second-look laparoscopy. Eighteen of these had no desire for pregnancy, 9 conceived before planned second-look laparoscopy and 5 were recommended in vitro fertilization (IVF) after EP surgery because of severe adhesions.

Both at EP surgery and at second-look laparoscopy, the anatomic conditions of the pelvis were registered on a preprinted form and lysis of adhesions was noted. At second-look laparoscopy tubal patency was tested by dye solution.

Results

Patients in the two groups did not differ with respect to gestational length, size and location of the gestation, estimated blood loss, preoperative serum hCG value, postoperative complications in terms of hematomas and second surgical interventions (Lundorff, et al., 1991b).

For each of the 73 woman a score change of the presence of adhesions between the primary operation and second-look laparoscopy could be calculated.

Presentation of the Adhesions

Laparoscopy group On the affected side, an impairment was noted in 5 patients (16%). 25 patients (81%) had an unchanged status and one patient (3%) had an improved status. On the contralateral side, 5 patients (16%) had an impaired status,

23 had an unchanged status (74%) and 3 had an improved status (10%).
Laparotomy group On the affected side, 22 patients (52%) had an impaired status, 18 patients (43%) had status quo and 2 patients (5%) were improved. On the contralateral side, 13 patients had impairment of the status (31%), 29 patients status quo (69%) and no patient improved the status.

Patients operated on by laparoscopy developed less adhesions than those patients treated by laparotomy. On the operated side the difference was statistically significant ($p<0.001$). No statistical significant difference was seen on the contralateral side.

Presentation of Tubal Status

There was no statistically significant difference between the surgical methods with regard to impairment of the score and improvements/status quo. In comparison between the surgical methods, improvements of the scores were classified as unchanged status, as improvement is a result of lysis of adhesions at primary surgery and not a consequence of the surgical method per se.

Tubal patency In the laparoscopy group the tube was patent in 76% and in the laparotomy group patency was found in 86%. There was no statistically significant difference between the two groups with regard to patency neither on the operated side nor on the contralateral side.

In this controlled trial we can demonstrate that the laparoscopic surgery in tubal pregnancy causes less adhesion formation on the operated side compared to conventional surgery. On the other hand, we found no statistical significant differences in adhesion formation on the contralateral side, in the tubal condition or in tubal patency. A possible explanation is that we, in case of laparotomy, used the Levinson and Swolin atraumatic technique, which can account for the favorable outcome in these patients. Nevertheless, we found that patients in the laparoscopy group develop substantial less adhesions compared to the laparotomy group, in spite of not using intraperitoneal lavage/rinsing with any solution of known anti-adhesion formation ability,

We conclude from this trial that adhesion formation occurs less frequently after laparoscopic treatment for tubal pregnancy compared to laparotomy using atraumatic technique. Whether this reduction of adhesion formation will increase the subsequent fertility remained to be evaluated by a life table analysis, using questionnaires to all 105 patients participating in the trial.

Fertility

Questionnaires including items such as wish for pregnancy and outcome, use of contraceptives during the study period and time "at risk" for pregnancy, were sent to all 105 patients one year after surgery and at the end of the study period (Lundorff, 1991c). 87 patients, 42 from the laparoscopy group and 45 from the laparotomy group, desired a pregnancy, and 50 conceived during the study period. Thirteen women were "at risk" for pregnancy < 18 months and 5 for > 30 months. Seventy percent of the first subsequent pregnancies occurred within one year of the "at risk" period, and 95% within 18 months. After 21 months "at risk," no further successful pregnancies were seen. Only EPs were observed after 28 months "at risk". The EP/IUP ratio increased parallel to the time "at risk."

Conception rates related to surgical methods The total conception rate in both surgical groups was just below 60% and the rate of first subsequent intrauterine pregnancy as well as the ratio of EP/IUP did not differ significantly between the two surgical methods.

Impacts of adhesions and adhesiolysis The possible importance of adhesions and adhesiolysis was further analyzed regardless of the treatment to which the patients belonged.

Forty-five of the 64 patients who underwent second-look laparoscopy after EP surgery had adhesions of varying degrees. The subsequent conception rate did not differ significantly between patients with or without adhesions. In patients without adhesions and with bilateral patency, intrauterine pregnancies were observed exclusively. Furthermore, both patients with contralateral patency and patients with bilateral patency had a higher frequency of intrauterine pregnancies. Among patients with only ipsilateral patency, the intrauterine pregnancy rate was significantly lower than in all other cases. Adhesiolysis was performed at second-look laparoscopy in 10 of 29 patients in the laparoscopy group and in 23 of 35 patients in the laparotomy group (NS).

Conclusion

In this investigation, the overall conception rate of < 60% is rather low. An explanation for this might be the short follow-up period. Our patients were "at risk" for pregnancy for an average of only 14 months. Thirteen patients were followed for < 18 months with no conception and some of these would probably have conceived if the follow-up period had been extended. Adhesiolysis at second look laparoscopy was performed in 24% of patients in the laparoscopy group and in 51% in the laparotomy group. The higher rate of adhesiolysis in the laparotomy group probably reflects on increased adhesion formation after laparotomy (Lundorff, et al., 1991a). Among all subsequent intrauterine pregnancies in the laparoscopy group, 18% had been subjected to adhesiolysis, versus 45% in the laparotomy group. To what extent the adhesiolysis has contributed to subsequent fertility is difficult to say as the adhesiolysis was not performed as a randomized trial.

According to the design of the study, the surgeons aim was to reestablish "normal anatomy" by adhesiolysis at a second-look laparoscopy. Complete adhesiolysis was achieved in 75% of cases. In the remaining cases, the adhesiolysis could not be successfully performed owing to anatomical and/or technical factors. This study thus shows that the prospects for fertility are similar in the laparoscopy and laparotomy group when a second-look laparoscopy with adhesiolysis is performed. It is possible that this adhesiolysis performed in half of the laparotomy cases compensate for the better adhesion scores after second-look laparoscopy and thus for more intrauterine pregnancies in this group.

REFERENCES

Bronson RA, Wallach EE (1977): Lysis of periadnexal adhesions for correction of infertility. Fertil Steril 28:613-9.

Bruhat MA, Manhes H, Mage G, Pouly JL (1980): Treatment of ectopic pregnancy by means of laparoscopy. Fertil Steril 33:411-4.

Caspi E, Halperin Y, Bukowsky I (1979): The importance of periadnexal adhesions in tubal reconstructive surgery for infertility. Fertil Steril 31:296-300.

DeCherney AH, Mezer HC (1984): The nature of posttuboplasty pelvic adhesions as determined by early and late laparoscopy. Fertil Steril 41:643.

Ellis H (1980): Internal overhealing: The problem of intraperitoneal adhesions. World J Surg 4:303-6.

Jansen RPS (1988): Early laparoscopy after pelvic operations to prevent adhesions: safety and efficacy. Fertil Steril 49:26-31.

Levinson CJ, Swolin K (1980): Postoperative adhesions: etiology, prevention and therapy. Clin Obstet Gynecol 23:1213-1220.

Lundorff P, Thorburn J, Lindblom B (1990): Second-look laparoscopy after ectopic pregnancy. Fertil Steril 53:604-609.

Lundorff P, Thorburn J, Hahlin M, Källfelt B, Lindblom B (1991a): Adhesion formation after laparoscopic surgery in tubal pregnancy : a randomized trial versus laparotomy. Fertil Steril 55:911-915.

Lundorff P, Thorburn J, Hahlin M, Källfelt B, Lindblom B (1991b): Short term benefits of laparoscopic surgery in ectopic pregnancy - a randomized trial versus laparotomy. Acta Obst Gynecol Scand 70:341-8.

Lundorff P, (1991c): Modern management of ectopic pregnancy. Early recognition, laparoscopic treatment and fertility prospects. Thesis (ISBN-91-628-0204-6), Göteburg, Sweden.

Mage G, Pouly J-L, Bouquet de Jolinière J, Chabrand S, Riouallon A, Bruhat M-A (1986): A preoperative classification to predict the intrauterine and ectopic pregnancy rates after tubal microsurgery. Fertil Steril 46:807-810.

Myhre-Jensen O, Larsen SB, Astrup T (1969): Fibrinolytic activity in serosal and synovial membranes. Archs Path 88:623-630.

Porter JM, McGregor FH, Mullen DC, Silver D (1969): Fibrinolytic activity of mesothelial surfaces. Surg Forum 20:80-82.

Pouly JL, Mahnes H, Mage G, Canis M, Bruhat MA (1986): Conservative laparoscopic treatment of 321 ectopic pregnancies. Fertil Steril 46:1093-1097.

Raftery AT (1981): Effect of peritoneal trauma on peritoneal fibrinolytic activity and intraperitoneal adhesion formation. Eur Surg Res 13:397-401.

Raj SG, Hulka JF (1982): Second-look laparoscopy in infertility surgery: therapeutic and prognostic value. Fertil Steril 38:325.

Rosenberg SM, Board JA (1983): Effectiveness of 32% high molecular weight dextran in reducing adhesions in human infertility surgery. Presented at the Thirtieth Annual Meeting of the Society for Gynecologic Investigation, March 17 to 20, Washington D.C.

Sherman D, Langer R, Sadovsky G, Bukovsky I, Caspi E (1982): Improved fertility following ectopic pregnancy. Fertil Steril 37:497-502.

Swolin K (1967): Die Einwirkung von grossen, intraperitonealen dosen Glucokortikoid auf die Bildung von postoperativen Adhäsionen. Acta Obstet Gynecol Scand 46.

Thorburn J, Berntsson C, Philipson M, Lindblom B (1986). Background factors of ectopic pregnancy. I. Frequency distribution in a case-control study. Eur J Gynecol Reprod Biol 23:321-331.

Thorburn J, Philipson M, Lindblom B (1988): Fertility after ectopic pregnancy in relation to background factors and surgical treatment. Fertil Steril 49: 595-601.

Trimbos-Kemper TCM, Trimbos JB, van Hall EV (1985): Adhesion formation after tubal surgery: results of the eighth-day laparoscopy in 188 patients. Fertil Steril 43:395.

Tuomivaara L, Kauppila A (1988): Radical or conservative surgery for ectopic pregnancy? A follow-up study of fertility of 323 patients. Fertil Steril 50:580-583.

Tulandi T, Collins JA, Burrows E, Jarrell JF, McInnes RA, Wrixon W, Simpson CW (1990). Treatment-dependent and treatment-independent pregnancy among women with periadnexal adhesions. Am J Obstet Gynecol 162:354-357.

Winston RML, Margara RA (1984): Conservative management of ectopic pregnancy. Obstet Gynecol 5:51-54.

Gynecologic Surgery and Adhesion Prevention, pages 149–153

EFFECTS OF RINGER'S LACTATE ON POSTSURGICAL ADHESION

Togas Tulandi, M.D.
Division of Reproductive Endocrinology and Infertility
Department of Obstetrics and Gynecology
McGill University
Montreal, Quebec, H3A 1A1, Canada

Reproductive surgery is still a frequent cause of adhesion formation. In attempts to decrease postsurgical adhesion formation, a wide variety of agents have been tested. These agents work either by decreasing the inflammatory response or by physical separation of raw surfaces. However, to date there are no proven agents that are unequivocally effective. In a clinical study evaluating the effects of glucocorticoids, promethazine, hyskon and heparin, Fayez and Schneider (1987) found that these substances have no therapeutic advantage over Ringer's lactate solution. This study, however, had no control group of untreated subjects. It is possible, therefore that none of these substances including Ringer's lactate instillation are effective in preventing adhesion formation. We recently evaluated the effects of Ringer's lactate, fibrin sealant (Tisseel, Immuno (Canada) Ltd, Vienna, Austria), INTERCEED(TC7) (Johnson and Johnson Medical, Inc., New Brunswick, NJ), Gore-Tex surgical membrane (W.L. Gore & Associates, Inc., Flagstaff, AZ) and amniotic membrane on postsurgical adhesion in a rat model.

ANIMAL MODEL

We used female Sprague Dawley white rats of reproductive age, weighing 225 to 250 grams as a model for postsurgical adhesion formation and reformation. Adhesions were induced by a standardized injury to the left uterine horn of each rat by denuding the serosa on the proximal antemesometric area with a scalpel until macroscopic punctate bleeding was seen and by electrocautery devascularization of that segment. The right uterine horn served as an internal control. Adhesion formation was evaluated 3 weeks after the initial surgery and the degree of adhesion was scored using an adhesion scoring scale. To evaluate adhesion reformation, adhesions were completely liberated at the second surgery and reformed adhesions were graded at a third laparotomy.

RINGER'S LACTATE INSTILLATION AND FIBRIN SEALANT

In our initial study, we compared the effects of Ringer's lactate instillation, fibrin sealant (Tisseel) and control (Caballero and Tulandi, in press). In Ringer's lactate group, Ringer's lactate solution was instilled into the abdominal cavity before abdominal closure and in Tisseel group, the denuded uterine horn was covered by fibrin sealant. The results showed that both Ringer's lactate instillation and fibrin sealant decreased adhesion formation, but the efficacy of fibrin sealant was not superior to that of Ringer's lactate instillation. Evaluation of adhesion reformation revealed that the degree of adhesion in the control group was significantly higher than in the Ringer's lactate group.

This preliminary study indicates that instillation of Ringer's lactate solution decreases adhesion formation and reformation. Although, the mechanism of action of Ringer's lactate instillation is not clear, it seems that the presence of high volume of Ringer's lactate in the abdominal cavity separates raw peritoneal surfaces and prevents adhesion formation. We found that Ringer's lactate is still found in the abdominal cavity of the rats 36 hours after instillation. It is also possible that solution of Ringer's lactate cleanses the newly formed fibrin exudate from the raw peritoneal surfaces. Fibrin exudate serves as a matrix for fibroblast and capillary formation. If not quickly removed by absorption or fibrinolysis, the initial fibrin deposition produces an inflammatory response, fibroblast proliferation and adhesion formation. This study also suggests that future studies evaluating the effects of a particular agent on adhesion formation should be compared to those of Ringer's lactate instillation.

RINGER'S LACTATE AND ADHESION BARRIERS

Currently, there are two commercially available adhesion barriers, Gore-Tex surgical membrane and INTERCEED(TC7). The efficacy of Gore-Tex, a thin sheet of expanded polytetrafluorethylene remains unclear. Golberg et al (1987) could not demonstrate its efficacy, but Boyers et al (1988) found that Gore-Tex decreases adhesion formation. INTERCEED(TC7) is an oxidized regenerated cellulose which has been shown to decrease adhesion formation in rabbits (Linsky et al, 1987; Diamond et al, 1991) and in a multicenter clinical study (INTERCEED Adhesion Barrier Study Group, 1989). We recently compared the efficacy of these barriers to Ringer's lactate instillation in a rat uterine horn model (Pagidas and Tulandi, In Press).

Confirming our previous observations, we found that Ringer's lactate instillation significantly decreases primary adhesion formation. Gore-Tex surgical membrane reduces adhesion formation, but its reduction is less than that of Ringer's lactate. The need for reoperation for removal of the membrane is an additional disadvantage.

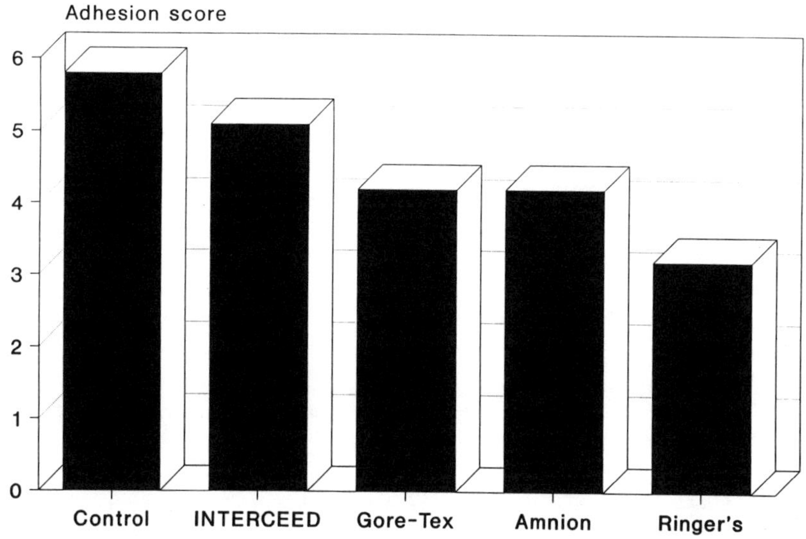

Figure I: Adhesion formation in the control rats and in rats which were treated with INTERCEED(TC7) adhesion barrier, Gore-Tex surgical membrane, amniotic membrane and Ringer's lactate instillation.

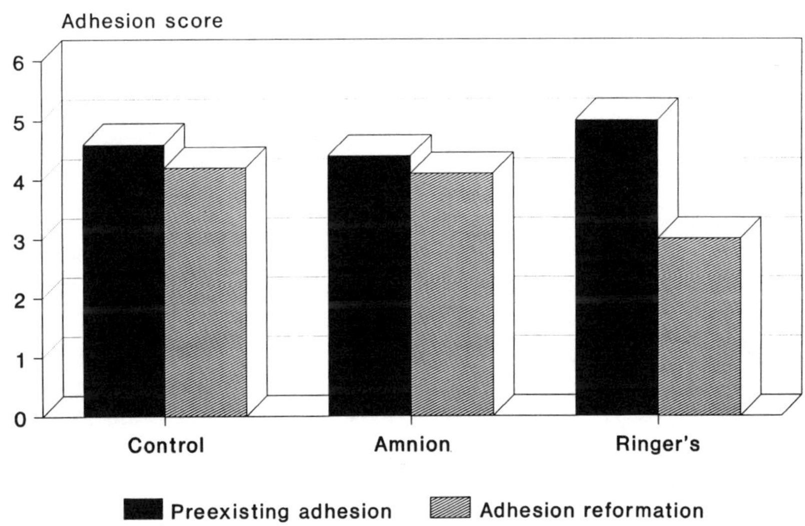

Figure II: Adhesion reformation in control rats and in rats which were treated with amniotic membrane graft and Ringer's lactate instillation.

Because of the inert property of Gore-Tex, perhaps it can be left in the abdominal cavity as a permanent implant. Contrary to previous studies in the rabbit horn scraping model (Linsky et al, 1987; Diamond et al, 1991), we found that in our rat model, no difference was found in the adhesion formation between the INTERCEED(TC7) group and the untreated control group. The addition of heparin does not change the results (Pagidas et al, submitted). It is possible that this is due to species difference and/or to the more extensive adhesions which we created by scraping and devascularization. Indeed, the ability of a substance or material to decrease adhesion formation is reduced if the adhesions are more extensive. In our animal model, Ringer's lactate instillation is superior to adhesion barriers (Figure I).

RINGER'S LACTATE AND AMNIOTIC MEMBRANE

The effects of amniotic membrane on adhesion formation is unclear. In the rat model, Badawy et al (1989) demonstrated no reduction in adhesion formation when applied to raw surfaces. Using trypsin treated amniotic graft, recently we confirmed the findings of Young et al (1991) that it is effective in reducing adhesion formation. Its efficacy, however is inferior to that of Ringer's lactate instillation. Furthermore, it reduces only adhesion formation but not reformation. Ringer's lactate instillation, on the other hand is effective in reducing both adhesion formation and reformation (Figure I and II).

CONCLUSION

Ringer's lactate instillation is widely used after a reproductive surgery. Its efficacy to decrease adhesion formation, however has never been demonstrated in human. In a rat model, it is effective in reducing adhesion formation and reformation and its efficacy is superior to that of the commercially available adhesion barriers and amniotic membrane (Figure I and II). Ringer's lactate is inexpensive, readily available and it has minimal side effects. Because of the beneficial effects of Ringer's lactate instillation on adhesion formation and reformation in a rat model, conditions required for an ethical randomized clinical trial would appear to exist. Future studies on the effects of various substances or materials on adhesion formation or reformation should be compared to Ringer's lactate instillation.

REFERENCES

Badawy SZ, Baggish MS, ElBakry MM, Baltoyiannis P (1989): Evaluation of tissue healing and adhesion formation after an intraabdominal amniotic membrane graft in the rat. J Reprod Med 34:198.

Boyers SP, Diamond MP, DeCherney AH (1988): Reduction of postoperative pelvic adhesions in the rabbit with Gore-Tex surgical membrane. Fertil Steril 49:1066-1070.

Caballero J, Tulandi T (In Press): Effects of Ringer's lactate and fibrin glue on postsurgical adhesions. J Reprod Med.

Diamond MP, Linsky CB, Cunningham T, Kamp L, Pines E, DeCherney AH, DiZerega GS (1991): Synergistic effects of INTERCEED (TC7) and heparin in reducing adhesion formation in the rabbit uterine horn model. Fertil Steril 55:389-394.

Diamond MP, Linsky CB, Cunningham T, Kamp L, Pines E, DeCherney AH, diZerega GS (1991): Adhesion reformation: Reduction by the use of INTERCEED(TC7) plus heparin. J Gynecol Surg 7:1-6.

Fayez JA, Schneider PJ (1987): Prevention of pelvic adhesion formation by different modalities of treatment. Am J Obstet Gynecol 157:1184-

Golberg JM. Toledo AA, Mitchell DE (1987): An evaluation of the Gore-Tex surgical membrane for the prevention of postoperative peritoneal adhesions. Obstet Gynecol 70:846-848.

INTERCEED(TC7) Adhesion Barrier Study Group (1989): Prevention of postsurgical adhesions by INTERCEED(TC7), an absorbable adhesion barrier: a prospective, randomized multicenter clinical study. Fertil Steril 51:933-938.

Linsky CB, Diamond MP, Constantine B et al (1987): Adhesion reduction in rabbit uerine horn model using an absorbable barrier, TC-7. J Reprod Med 32:17-19.

Pagidas K and Tulandi T: Effects of Ringer's lactate, INTERCEED(TC7) and Gore-Tex surgical membrane on postsurgical adhesions formation. Fertil Steril (In Press).

Pagidas K, Khalifa F and Tulandi T: Effects of Ringer's lactate, INTERCEED(TC7) plus heparin and amniotic membrane on adhesion formation and reformation (Submitted).

Young RL, Cota J, Zund G, Mason BA, Wheeler JM (1991): The use of an amniotic membrane graft to prevent postoperative adhesions. Fertil Steril 55:624-628.

Gynecologic Surgery and Adhesion Prevention, pages 155–185

MYOMECTOMY, GnRH ANALOGS, AND ADHESIONS

G. David Adamson, M.D., F.R.C.S.C., F.A.C.O.G., F.A.C.S.
Clinical Associate Professor
Department of Gynecology and Obstetrics
Stanford University School of Medicine
Stanford, CA 94305

Director, Fertility and Reproductive Health Institute of Northern California
San Jose, CA 95124

INTRODUCTION

Uterine fibroids is a common female medical problem, and surgery is often recommended for management. Recently, gonadotropin-releasing hormone (GnRH) agonists have been investigated for use in uterine fibroid disease, but many questions remain about their role in overall management. In addition, the impact of GnRH agonist use prior to myomectomy on the subsequent formation of adhesions is largely unknown. Since adhesions are a common and often important complication of myomectomy, the potential benefits of GnRH agonist use prior to myomectomy merits further clinical evaluation.

UTERINE FIBROIDS

Leiomyomas or uterine fibroids are the most common solid tumor of the female genital tract. Uterine leiomyomas are neoplasms of the smooth muscle and are benign, being found in about 20% of women over the age of 30 years (Healy, et al., 1986). Thus, therapeutic intervention is not always required. Indications for the treatment of uterine myomas include menorrhagia with iron deficiency anemia, uterine pressure or pain, rapidly increasing fibroid size, recurrent abortion with endometrial cavity distortion, and infertility with endometrial cavity distortion. Unexplained or refractory infertility may also be an indication for myomectomy (Coddington, et al.,1986).

At this time there is no effective permanent medical treatment for uterine fibroids. Rather, management of symptomatic fibroid patients has been surgical, either myomectomy or hysterectomy. Of the 650,000 hysterectomies performed annually in the United States, approximately 27% or 175,000 are performed for uterine myomas (DHEW publication no. (PHS) 88-1753). Myomectomy is performed in about 18,000 patients per year. Myomectomy has a recurrence rate of approximately 15% (range, 4% to 59%) and a repeat operation rate of approximately 10% (range, 3% to 21%), and subsequent hysterectomy is required in an additional 1% to 5% of patients (Malone, 1969) (Berkeley, et al., 1983).

Although the pathogenesis of myomas is not well established, it has been recognized that fibroid growth and maintenance are stimulated by estrogen and are affected by hormonal cyclic changes (Friedman, et al., 1990). Estrogen and progesterone receptors have been identified in myomatous tissue (Tamaya, et al., 1985). Because leiomyomas can be influenced by changes at the estrogen and progesterone receptors, GnRH agonists have been investigated as a potential treatment.

Several pilot and small studies have been reported in which GnRH agonists were evaluated for the treatment of uterine fibroids (Filicori, et al., 1983), (Maheux, et al., 1984), (Coddington, et al., 1986), (Healy, et al., 1986), (Lumsden, et al., 1987), (Friedman, et al., 1989a). Potential benefits of GnRH agonist therapy are a reduction in uterine fibroid size and uterine volume, decreased preoperative and perioperative blood loss, and an improvement in operative conditions. These potential benefits offer the possibility of reduced adhesion formation following myomectomy.

EFFECT OF GnRH AGONISTS ON FIBROID SIZE

A primary effect of GnRH agonists is to decrease uterine fibroid size. In Andreyko's study the effect of daily administration of nafarelin on uterine and myoma size was evaluated in 10 patients with the use of magnetic resonance imaging (Andreyko, et al., 1988). After six months of treatment, the size of the largest myoma decreased by a mean of 46% from baseline in 9 of 10 women. Uterine volume decreased by an average of 57% in all treated patients. Of note, both small and large myomas responded to nafarelin therapy but, consistent with other trials, myomas became enlarged again in several women after discontinuation of nafarelin.

In a more recent trial, Costantini et al. compared the effects of six months of treatment with intranasal buserelin or subcutaneous goserelin on myoma size (Costantini, et al., 1990). A reduction of more than 30% in myoma volume was seen in 34 of 42 (81%) patients, and no difference was seen between the two GnRH agonists (Fig. 1). As reported in other clinical trials, regrowth of the myomas followed the discontinuation of therapy (Friedman, et al., 1989b).

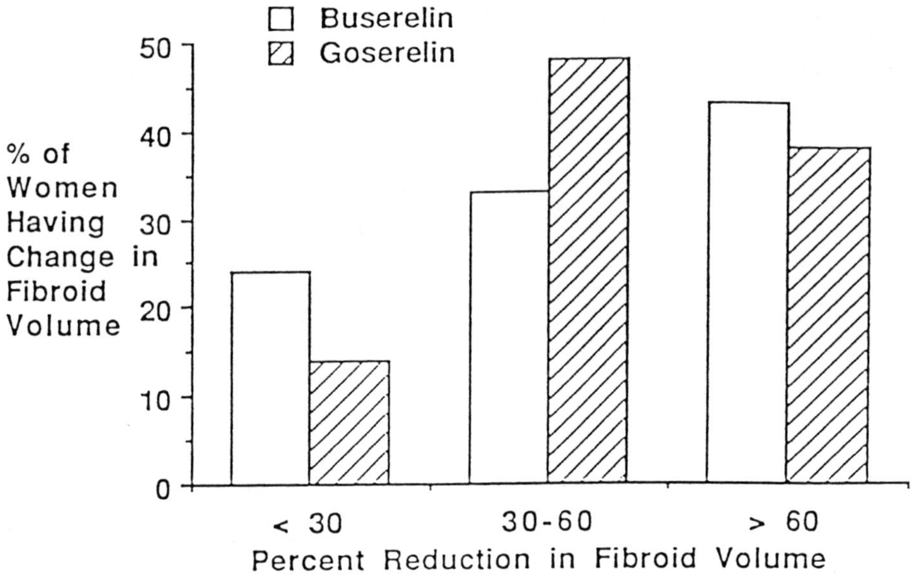

Fig. 1. Proportion of women having a change in fibroid volume from baseline to 6 months after treatment with buserelin (n=21) or goserelin (n=21). (Modified from Costantini et al. Eur J Obstet Gynecol Reprod Biol 1990;37:63-9).

One of the largest GnRH agonist trials was a multicenter, randomized, placebo-controlled trial in which the effects of intranasal nafarelin on menstrual blood loss and uterine and fibroid volume were evaluated in 166 patients scheduled for elective hysterectomy (Ylikorkala, 1990). Patients scheduled for hysterectomy for non-malignant conditions, including uterine fibroids, menorrhagia, or pelvic pain, were evaluated by ultrasound examination. Patients were randomized in a 2:1 ratio to treatment with either intranasal nafarelin, 200 ug twice daily, or placebo for 3 months or until hysterectomy. In patients with fibroids, the total volume of the three largest fibroids decreased by 31% from admission to 3 months in the nafarelin group but increased by 1.2% in the placebo group (p=0.024; Fig. 2). Assessment of the largest fibroid at the time of surgery suggested a decrease in the volume of the largest fibroid with nafarelin compared with placebo, but the difference was not statistically significant (p=0.055).

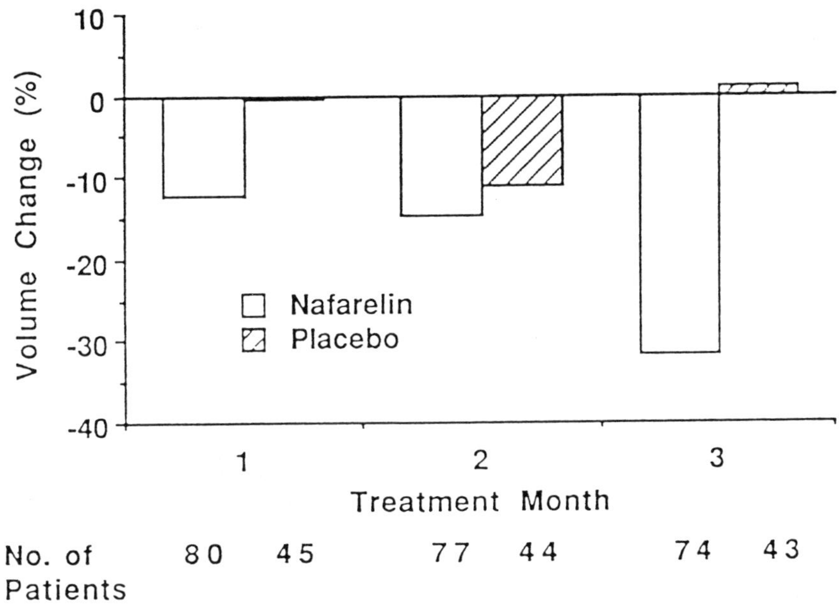

Fig. 2. Median percentage change in volume of the largest three fibroids (Ylikorkala, 1990). P=0.024 for nafarelin vs. placebo by two-way analysis Of variance.

Reproduced from *Treatment of Uterine Fibroids: New Findings with GnRH Analogs* Am J Obstet Gynecol 1992:164(2) with permission from Mosby-Yearbook, Inc.

All GnRH agonist studies to date have shown a variable but significant decrease in myoma size; however, myomas almost always return to pretreatment size after discontinuation of therapy. The reasons for this response within a few months to GnRH agonist therapy have been studied. Pasqualini et al. evaluated the effect of the GnRH agonist decapeptyl on hormone levels and receptors in uterine myomas and found that myoma tissue was very sensitive to changes in hormone levels (Pasqualini, et al., 1990). This occurs because myoma tissue has receptors for estrogen and progesterone and thus is affected by both cyclic changes in hormone levels and pharmacologic therapy such as GnRH agonists, which alter hormonal levels (Marugo, et al., 1989). The number of estrogen receptors is greatest during the follicular phase and decreases during the post-ovulatory phase. Further, estrogen and progesterone receptors are more numerous in submucous than subserosal myomas. This has led to the hypothesis that submucous myomas may respond better to GnRH agonist therapy than large subserosal myomas. In addition, the effect of GnRH agonists on myomas is to decrease cell size and intracellular matrix but not the number of cells. The histopathologic appearance of fibroids also does not change with leuprolide treatment (Gutmann, et al., 1991). Therefore it is not surprising that myomas return to pretreatment size after GnRH agonists are discontinued.

EFFECT OF GnRH AGONISTS ON UTERINE SIZE

GnRH agonists also decrease uterine size (Andreyko, et al., 1988). In a prospective randomized trial, Friedman et al. demonstrated a reduction in uterine volume with leuprolide acetate (Friedman, et al., 1989b). Eighteen women were randomly assigned to receive monthly intramuscular injections of leuprolide or placebo for 24 weeks. A significant ($p<0.05$) reduction in uterine volume at 12 and 24 weeks compared with pretreatment volume was noted in the leuprolide group (Fig. 3).

However, uterine volume returned to 88% of pretreatment levels by 3 months after discontinuation of GnRH therapy. Others have confirmed this reduction in uterine volume (Nakamura, et al., 1991). The reduction in uterine volume achieved with agonists is counteracted if medroxyprogesterone acetate is given at the same time (Friedman, et al., 1988).

In another large double-blind multicenter trial, leuprolide or placebo were administered to 128 women with leiomyomata uteri every 4 weeks for 24 weeks (Friedman, et al., 1991). Mean uterine volume decreased by 45% in patients treated with leuprolide compared with a 5% increase in those given placebo. Uterine volume returned to pretreatment size by 24 weeks after leuprolide was stopped.

Another study using nafarelin showed that both the length and volume of the myomatous uteri were decreased significantly ($p<0.05$) in the nafarelin group compared with the placebo group (Ylikorkala, 1990). These findings were confirmed during surgery when the uterine weight was measured. There was a significant decrease in uterine weight in the nafarelin group compared with the placebo group in all patients and in patients with fibroids only.

It is clear from numerous well designed studies that GnRH agonists reduce both uterine and myoma size approximately by half. However, this effect is variable from patient to patient, from myoma to myoma in the same patient, and myomas return to their original size within a few months of discontinuing treatment.

OTHER CLINICAL EFFECTS OF GnRH TREATMENT OF UTERINE FIBROIDS

Other clinical effects of pre-operative GnRH agonist treatment of uterine fibroids include a reduction in menstrual blood loss. In one study,

55% of patients with severe blood loss at baseline randomly assigned to nafarelin therapy had no bleeding after 3 months compared with 10% of the placebo-treated patients ($P<0.001$) (Ylikorkala, 1990). In contrast, only 14% of patients receiving nafarelin continued to have severe menstrual bleeding at the end of therapy compared with only 48% of placebo patients (Fig. 4). Additionally, a mean increase of 4.2% in hemoglobin levels was noted before surgery in patients treated with nafarelin compared with a decrease of 2.7% in the placebo group ($P=0.032$).

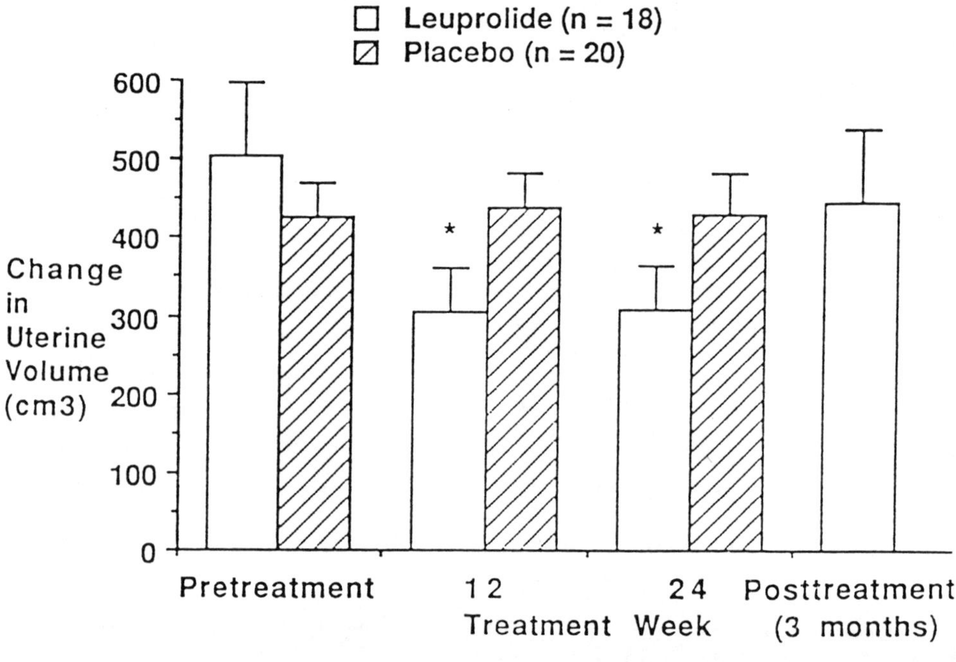

Fig. 3. Change in uterine volume (mean+/- standard error) during treatment with depot leuprolide acetate or placebo in women with uterine fibroids. $P<0.05$ vs. pretreatment by the Dunnett *t* test.

Reproduced from *Treatment of Uterine Fibroids: New Findings with GnRH Analogs* Am J Obstet Gynecol 1992:164(2) with permission from Mosby-Yearbook, Inc.

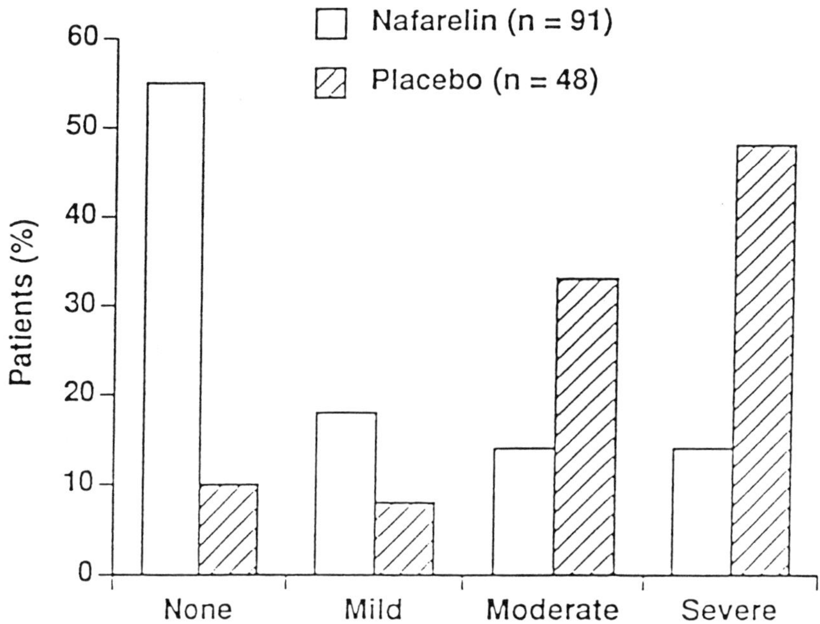

Fig. 4. Severity of menstrual blood loss at 3 months in women treated with nafarelin or placebo before elective hysterectomy (Ylikorkala, 1990). P<0.001 for nafarelin vs. placebo by Cochran-Mantel-Haenszel test.

In another study, patients were treated with 3.6 mg. of subcutaneous goserelin every 28 days for 6 months (Lumsden, et al., 1987). In addition to a reduction in myoma and uterine size, there was a reduction in menstrual blood loss. Similar findings were reported in a large leuprolide study (Friedman, et al., 1991). In addition, symptoms improved in most patients and 37 of 38 patients (97%) with menorrhagia at baseline had resolution by the end of treatment.

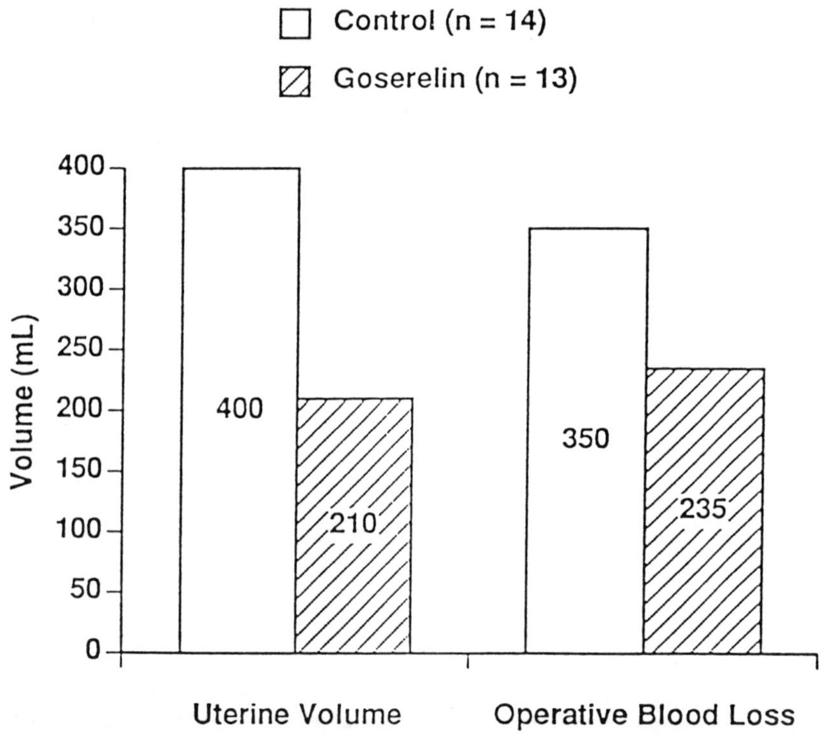

Fig. 5. Uterine volume and operative blood loss in women with symptomatic uterine fibroids treated for 3 months before elective hysterectomy. P<0.01 for goserelin vs. placebo by Wilcoxon two-sample test.

Reproduced from *Treatment of Uterine Fibroids: New Findings with GnRH Analogs* Am J Obstet Gynecol 1992:164(2) with permission from Mosby-Yearbook, Inc.

Shaw has reported a reduction in blood loss at myomectomy, Lumsden at hysterectomy (Fig. 5), and Ylikorkala at hysterectomy (Lumsden, et al., 1987), (Shaw, 1989), (Ylikorkala, 1990). Friedman, however, showed a significant reduction in total intraoperative blood loss only in patients treated with leuprolide acetate depot with uterine volume greater than 600 cm^3 before treatment (Friedman, et al., 1989a). Matta showed a reduction in uterine blood flow with GnRH agonist use (Matta, et al., 1988).

The decrease in vaginal bleeding and resultant increase in hemoglobin and hematocrit, as well as the reduced intraoperative blood loss have several potential benefits, although it must be emphasized that prospective randomized studies proving these potential benefits have not yet been performed. The patient's hematocrit level may be sufficient to allow her to give autologous blood donations before surgery. This and the lessened perioperative blood loss may reduce the need for blood transfusion and/or hysterectomy at the time of surgery. Risks associated with blood transfusion, which are often overlooked or underestimated, may be reduced. Between 8% and 18% of patients require blood or blood products at surgery; the current risk of hepatitis is approximately 8% per transfusion (Dicker, et al., 1982), (Berkeley, et al., 1983), (Koziol, et al., 1986). Other potential advantages from the use of GnRH agonists may result from a reduction of uterine myoma size. These include the use of more conservative surgery; that is, the condition may be managed with myomectomy rather than hysterectomy or endoscopically. Smaller and fewer incisions may result in decreased tissue trauma and increased preservation of normal tissue. Other potential advantages are listed in Table 1.

Table 1. POTENTIAL ADVANTAGES OF A REDUCTION IN UTERINE AND MYOMA SIZE BY GnRH AGONISTS

Reduced vascularity
* Reduced menorrhagia
* Increased hematocrit and iron
* Autologous donation
* Less operative blood loss
* Reduced risk of blood transfusion
* Reduced risk of hepatitis

Operative technique
* Hysterectomy less likely
* Operative laparoscopy more likely
* Fewer, smaller incisions
* Less tissue trauma
* Less risk of injury
* Pfannenstiel incision more feasible
* Vaginal hysterectomy more feasible

Integrity of uterine cavity
* Hysteroscopic approach
* Avoidance of uterine cavity at laparotomy

IMPLICATIONS OF GnRH TREATMENT OF UTERINE FIBROIDS ON ADHESION FORMATION

Numerous factors contribute to adhesion formation (Rosenberg, 1990) (Drollette, 1992). These include tissue trauma which can be reduced by gentle tissue handling, avoidance of exposure to air, and avoidance of drying by constant irrigation and shorter operating times. Infection can also cause adhesion formation, but its risk can be reduced by the use of prophylactic antibiotics. Ischemia is a major cause of adhesions, but can be reduced by not placing the tissue on tension with sutures.

De-peritonealized surfaces will regenerate a new serosal layer if other pelvic structures do not contact the fibrin mesh on the de-peritonealized surface. Methods used to attempt to keep the surfaces apart include round ligament suspension, use of fluids to float tissues and adhesion barriers.

Hemorrhage can facilitate adhesion formation when the fibrin clot provides a matrix for invasion by fibroblasts. Use of magnification and bipolar cautery can reduce oozing, as can avoidance of aspirin and non-steroidal anti-inflammatory drugs for several weeks prior to surgery.

Techniques for hemostasis include the injection of a dilute solution of vasopressin into the base of the myoma. It is also important to control bleeding quickly at laparoscopy because bleeding which would ordinarily be insignificant at laparotomy can quickly obscure the surgeon's view, resulting potentially in the need for laparotomy or transfusion. Hemostasis can also be improved by coagulating and/or isolating a vessel prior to cutting it. Hemostasis may be facilitated by use of the CO_2 laser and also fiber lasers. The microbipolar and Kleppinger forceps should also be available at all times. The maintenance of hemostasis will increase the surgeon's ability to perform the surgery without using clips, staples, sutures or Roeder loops which are foreign bodies which can increase adhesion formation. Foreign bodies such as suture should also be used as little as possible since these have been shown to be associated with adhesion formation (Nezhat, et al., 1991).

Myomectomy at laparotomy has been documented to result in adhesion formation (Berkeley, et al., 1983). Patients in Berkeley's study who did not conceive had larger myomas than those who did conceive, but this group also had a greater number of myomas, and the cavity was entered more often, making it difficult to draw firm conclusions from the results. However, of six patients with only myomas as a presumed cause of infertility, only one conceived. Four of the remaining five had second-look laparoscopy and all had significant peritubal adhesions which had not been present at the time of the first procedure. This strongly suggests that adhesion formation is a common sequelae of myomectomy and that these adhesions may have a significant deleterious effect on fertility. Studies have confirmed the deleterious effect of adhesions on fertility (Tulandi, et al., 1990), (Fig. 6). Malone found that patients with multiple fibroid tumors were less likely to conceive and carry to term than those with a single fibroid and were more likely to require future definitive surgical treatment (Malone, 1969). Taken together these studies suggest that careful consideration needs to be given to the indications for myomectomy in the woman still desiring fertility and that it is important to make attempts to reduce adhesion formation.

EFFECT OF SALPINGOOVARIOLYSIS
ON PREGNANCY RATE

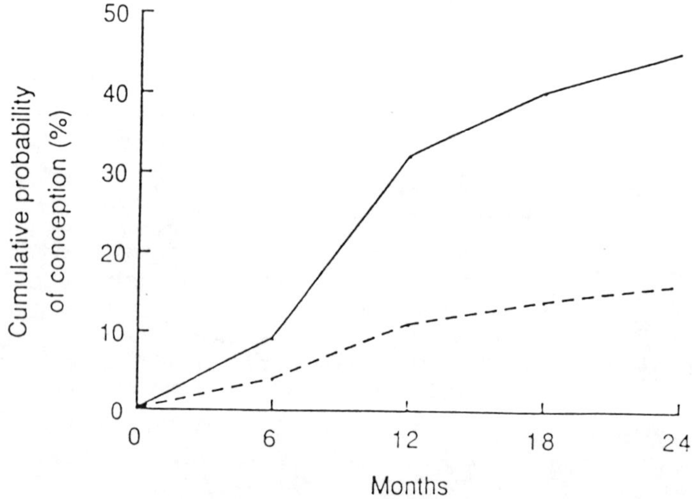

Fig. 6. Cumulative probability of conception among women with periadnexal adhesions who were treated by salpingoovariolysis (*solid line*) and who were not treated (*broken line*). (Tulandi et al. (1990)

Reproduced from *Treatment of Uterine Fibroids: New Findings with GnRH Analogs* Am J Obstet Gynecol 1992:164(2) with permission from Mosby-Yearbook, Inc.

Studies by Diamond et al. show that adhesions reform 50-90% of the time following laparotomy for adhesiolysis when adjuvant methods are not used (Interceed (TC7) Adhesion Barrier Study Group, 1989). Other data show that at least some adhesions formed in 96% of patients following laparoscopic surgery, but that de novo adhesions do not form as frequently as those at laparotomy (Diamond, et al., 1990).

Perez also showed a 66% recurrence rate following laparotomy adhesiolysis in both adhesions and endometriosis patients (Perez, 1991). He felt that second-look laparoscopy was beneficial since only 47% of those undergoing third-look laparoscopy had adhesions. He also felt laparotomy microsurgical techniques might result in fewer adhesions than laparoscopic treatment.

Dunn found at second-look laparoscopy that adhesions reformed at 56% of the initially lysed sites after laparoscopy and that de novo adhesion formation occurred at 23% of sites (Dunn, 1991). He felt this de novo adhesion reformation may be less than the generally reported half of all laparotomy patients. Fewer adhesions also occurred following laparoscopic compared with laparotomy treatment of ectopic pregnancy (Lundorff, et al., 1991). Animal studies also suggest less adhesion formation following laparoscopy compared to laparotomy (Luciano, et al., 1989), (Das, et al., 1990). Other animal studies suggest that even barrier methods may have limited efficacy in reducing adhesion formation (Pagidas, Tulandi, 1992), (Haney, Doty, 1992).

Laparoscopic myomectomy has been reported by Nezhat in 154 women with fibroids ranging from 3 to 15 cm. in size (Nezhat, et al., 1991). Seventy-seven women with a history of menometrorrhagia and anemia, or with leiomyomata larger than 5 cm. on ultrasonography were treated with leuprolide acetate preoperatively for one to four months. The serosal edges of myomas less than 3 cm. were reapproximated with the bipolar coagulator while those larger were initially reapproximated with interrupted plain catgut suture and later 4-0 PDS (polydioxanone) endosuture. Defects in broad ligaments were not closed. After excision, myomas were removed either intact or in pieces via posterior colpotomy, through suprapubic anterior wall incisions or through the operating channel of the laparoscope or accessory instrument.

Two women received blood transfusions. Twenty-eight women had second-look laparoscopy and four subsequently had laparotomy. The sites of pedunculated and superficial subserosal leiomyomata had healed completely. At the sites of 37 intramural and deep subserosal leiomyomata which were removed without suturing the myometrium there was evidence of granulation and all sites showed indentation of the uterus. The depth of indentation was directly proportional to the size of the leiomyoma. These indentations probably represent structural defects in the uterus. Sutured sites of intramural or deep subserosal leiomyomata healed more completely than the unsutured sites but were associated with a greater incidence of adhesion formation. Adhesions formed more frequently when the myoma was posterior compared to the fundal and anterior portion of the uterus. Among the 56 myomectomy sites evaluated, both the incidence and severity of adhesion formation were greater at sutured sites of leiomyomata > 3cm. than at any of the unsutured sites. (Table 2).

Nezhat et al. concluded that multiple and large myomata were more difficult to excise, resulted in more bleeding and were more cumbersome and time-consuming to remove from the uterine cavity. Pedunculated myomas were the easiest to excise and remove. Subserosal and intramural myomas, depending on the size and depth of penetration required more skill, manipulation and care to avoid bleeding and risk to other organs. Removal of the myoma was the most time-consuming part of the procedure, and except in the case of calcified myomas, was dependent on the size of the myoma. The need to remove the myomas via colpotomy or mini-laparotomy increased surgical time, risk of infection, injury to other organs, and length of recovery. Suturing was required more frequently for larger myomas to prevent large indentations, but also resulted in more adhesions.

Table 2. INCIDENCE OF ADHESION FORMATION AND GRADE AFTER LAPAROSCOPIC MYOMECTOMY AT 56 SITES DURING SECOND-LOOK LAPAROSCOPY OR LAPAROTOMY

SIZE OF LEIO-MYOMA	NO SUTURE USED				SUTURE USED			
	ADHESION GRADE				ADHESION GRADE			
	0	1	2	3	0	1	2	3
<3 CM	18/21	3/21	0/21	0/21	N/A	N/A	N/A	N/A
>3 CM	10/16	5/16	1/16	0/16	0/19	4/19	12/19	5/19

GRADES OF ADHESIONS: 0=NO ADHESIONS; 1=FILMY AND NON-VASCULAR; 2=THICK AND NONVASCULAR; 3=THICK, VASCULAR, AND BOWEL.

ADAPTED FROM NEZHAT ET AL. (1991), INT J FERTIL 36:278.

Dubuisson et al. performed six laparotomies and 43 laparoscopies for myomectomy (Dubuisson, et al, 1991). Follow-up laparoscopy performed six weeks after the initial laparoscopy in six cases showed no adhesions in five cases and severe bowel adhesions to the myomectomy scar in one patient. Dubuisson et al. concluded that preoperative treatment with GnRH agonists may be beneficial by facilitating surgery, reducing uterine blood flow, and reducing operative blood loss. They now routinely use GnRH agonists preoperatively.

Several authors have emphasized that myomectomy should be an atraumatic procedure which minimizes blood loss (Smith, Uhlir, 1990), (Berkeley, et al., 1983), (Rosenfeld, 1986). It is generally felt also that if equivalent procedures can be performed at laparoscopy or hysteroscopy, the endoscopic approach is preferred to laparotomy (Adamson, 1992), (Adamson, 1991), (Operative Laparoscopy Study Group, 1991), (Peterson, et al., 1990), (Levine, 1985), (Vietz, 1989).

GnRH AGONIST INFLUENCE ON THE ENDOCRINOLOGY AND IMMUNOLOGY OF ADHESION FORMATION

Heinonin (1990) has suggested that peritoneal fluid leukotriene B4 and prostaglandin E_2, which are higher in women with acute salpingitis, may play a role in development of peritoneal adhesions. Thompson (1989) has reported that inflamed peritoneum had less and visceral ischemia resulted in less plasminogen activator activity. Vipond also found that plasminogen activator activity was lower in inflamed peritoneum than control tissue (Vipond, 199). It is possible that GnRH agonist use might reduce the degree of inflammation associated with other disease such as infection or endometriosis pre-operatively, or the amount of inflammation post-operatively. Such a reduction in inflammation could theorectically reduce ultimate adhesion formation. de Ziegler (deZiegler, 1991) showed that at physiological levels of estradiol decreased vascular resistance of uterine arteries. It is probable the hypoestrogenism resulting from

GnRH agonist use would alter vascular resistance, thereby affecting pelvic blood flow and possibly altering the immune response. Whether or not this would be beneficial is still conjecture. GnRH agonists use has also been shown to reduce the growth-hormone releasing hormone-stimulated growth hormone release, and has been shown to affect insulin-like growth factor-I and TSH (Word, 1990). The possibility exists that these hormone changes could alter adhesion formation.

Patients who have endometriosis concomitantly with fibroids might also benefit from pre-operative GnRH agonist use. Henzl (Henzl, 1988) has shown that lesions are reduced, possibly resulting in less inflammatory stimulation in the pelvis. It is also clear that endometriosis lesions stimulate an immune response.(Mathur, 1990, Badawy, 1989, Homm, 19889)

Reduction of the endometriosis lesion activity by GnRH agonist use should result in a decreased immunological response. Since this immunological response over a prolonged period of time is known to result in adhesions associated with endometriosis, it is possible that reduction of this response might reduce the risk of adhesions forming over a shorter interval post-myomectomy.

DISADVANTAGES OF GnRH AGONIST THERAPY

Treatment with GnRH agonists is not benign. The well known hypoestrogenic side effects include hot flashes and bone loss (Friedman, 1990), (Henzl, 1988). In addition, about 2% of patients receiving GnRH agonist therapy can experience a very profuse vaginal hemorrhage requiring immediate surgical management (Thorp, Katz, 1991). This serious clinical problem has been reported to date only in patients with submucous myomas. The cause of this adverse event is thought to be a reduction in myoma size and a loss of mechanical compression of the vessels within the uterus. Also, painful fibroid degeneration may occur.

Some investigators have been concerned that myomas may be reduced to an undetectable size by pre-operative GnRH agonist use. Results from a recent trial of buserelin before myomectomy suggested that this phenomenon occurs (Fedele, et al., 1990). In this randomized trial, a 44% decrease in uterine volume was observed during buserelin therapy in eight patients compared with no change in 16 untreated control patients. Intraoperative blood loss and postoperative morbidity did not differ between groups. However, at the 6-month post-operative evaluation, only 2 of 16 (13%) patients in the untreated group had myomas smaller than 1.5 cm. in size compared with 5 of 8 (63%) patients in the buserelin group. These data suggest that small myomas may have been missed at the time of surgery because of pre-operative treatment with buserelin. The results of this study need to be confirmed by others, and if true, its clinical relevance established.

GnRH ANTAGONISTS COMPARED WITH AGONISTS

GnRH antagonists are currently being investigated in animals and early human trials. Their major advantage is the ability to cause immediate down regulation and desensitization of the receptors so that the initial "flare" reaction of increased gonadotropins and estradiol levels does not occur. This allows the antagonist to achieve immediate estradiol suppression at the initiation of treatment. The clinical benefit potentially is avoidance of fibroid stimulation, and potentially a shorter duration of treatment. Unfortunately, side effects of the antagonists, in particular those related to histamine release, severely limit their current clinical application. Expectations are that within approximately six to eight years newer, improved antagonists will become available for general clinical use.

STRATEGIES FOR MANAGING UTERINE MYOMAS

Despite promising results of GnRH agonist therapy of uterine fibroids, surgery remains the only effective long-term treatment. Several different procedures are appropriate including myomectomy by either laparoscopy, laparotomy, or hysteroscopy or hysterectomy abdominally, vaginally, or with laparoscopically-assisted vaginal hysterectomy. However, the use of GnRH agonists as preoperative adjuncts has some potential benefits. Preoperative use may increase the feasibility of performing myomectomy instead of hysterectomy, increase the use of laparoscopic, hysteroscopic, or vaginal procedures, preserve normal uterine tissue, facilitate the operative technique, and reduce blood loss. These potential benefits may have significant impact on reducing adhesion formation by reducing tissue trauma, infection, ischemia, denuded surface areas, hemorrhage and the exposure to foreign bodies such as starch granules, sponges, sutures, clips and staples. The choice of therapy will depend on the surgical aspects of treatment, but also on the size and number of myomata, the age of the patient, and the desire to preserve fertility and uterine function (Table 3).

Table 3. POTENTIAL BENEFITS OF PREOPERATIVE GnRHa ON ADHESION FORMATION FOLLOWING MYOMECTOMY

Causes of Adhesion Formation	Potential Benefits of GnRHa
Tissue Trauma	* Smaller incisions * Fewer incisions * Decreased tissue dissection * Decreased bleeding in tissue * Hysterectomy less likely * Laparoscopic/hysteroscopic approach more likely * Avoidance of uterine cavity at laparotomy * Shorter operating time with smaller myomas

(Continued)

Infection	* Endoscopic or vaginal approach more likely * Decreased tissue dissection * Shorter operating time with smaller myomas
Ischemia	* Decreased sutures with smaller myomas * Decreased need for coagulation * Decreased tissue dissection * Decreased operative blood loss * Availability of autologous donation
Denuded Surface Apposition	* Decreased tissue dissection * Better visualization, decreased tissue manipulation * Fewer incisions * Smaller incisions * Hysteroscopic approach
Foreign Body	* Decreased need for sutures * Laparoscopic/hysteroscopic approach * Decreased operative blood loss
Hemorrhage	* Decreased dissection * Decreased bleeding * Reduced operating time * Better visualization * Laparoscopic/hysteroscopic approach
Endocrine/Immune Response	* Reduced peritoneal inflammation * Reduced vascular flow * Reduced growth hormone * Reduced concomitant endometriosis

One innovative strategy for managing uterine fibroids with medical therapy only is to combine the GnRH agonist with an estrogen-progestin combination. In a preliminary trial, five women with leiomyomata uteri were treated with leuprolide for 24 weeks (Friedman, 1989c). After 3 months, conjugated estrogens were added on days 1 to 25 and medroxyprogesterone acetate from days 16 to 25. Patients were followed for as long as 2 years. A 49% decrease in uterine volume was seen at 3 months, but no further decrease was seen during the next 2 years. There was also a decrease in vasomotor symptoms, and bone density was preserved. These results were encouraging, but additional data obtained on more patients and a longer duration of study have shown a regrowth of the myomas in some patients taking this regimen (Friedman, personal communication). This confirms not only that leiomyomata and myometrium are estrogen sensitive, but suggests that an estrogenic threshold exists for uterine growth (Friedman, 1990; Barbieri, 1991). It can be seen that different treatment strategies that use GnRH agonists show promise, but the optimal approach to medical treatment of uterine fibroids is unclear. Further studies, many currently ongoing, will help us understand how to use GnRH agonists better in the future.

CONCLUSION

Results from clinical trials have consistently shown the efficacy of GnRH agonists as a pre-operative adjunct for reducing myoma and uterine size and pre-operative and perioperative blood loss. Uterine myomas are very sensitive to hormonal changes which are probably mediated through estrogen and progesterone receptors. This impact on fibroid receptors is the most likely mechanism by which GnRH agonists can effect changes in myomas. Despite these effects the role of GnRH agonists in the management of uterine myomas has not yet been fully defined. However, their use as a presurgical adjunct appears to facilitate myomectomy and preservation of healthy uterine tissue. These intraoperative benefits can reasonably be expected, but are not yet proven, to reduce adhesion formation, a common and clinically significant sequelae of myomectomy.

REFERENCE LIST

Adamson GD, Subak LL, Pasta DJ, Hurd SJ, vonFranque O, Rodriguez BA (1992): Comparison of CO_2 laser laparoscopy with laparotomy for treatment of endometriomata. Fertil Steril 57(5):965-73.

Adamson GD (1991): The choice of medical therapy for the operative treatment of endometriosis is endoscopic laser surgery. Contemp Obstet Gynecol 7:129-31.

Andreyko JL, Blumenfeld Z, Marshall LA, Monroe SE, Hricak H, Jaffe RB (1988): Use of an agonistic analog of gonadotropin-releasing hormone (nafarelin) to treat leiomyomas: assessment by magnetic resonance imaging. Am J Obstet Gynecol 158:903-10.

Badawy SZA, Cuenca V, Kaufman L, Stitzel A, Thompson M (1989): The regulation of immunoglobulin production by B cells in patients with endometriosis. Fertil Steril 51:770-773.

Barbieri RL, Gordon AMC (1991): Hormonal therapy of endometriosis: the estradiol target. Fertil Steril 56:820-22.

Berkeley AS, DeCherney AH, Polan ML (1983): Abdominal myomectomy and subsequent fertility. Surg Gynecol Obstet 156:319-24.

Best CL, Rittenhouse D, Sueldo C (1991): A comparison of TC7 and 32% dextran 70 for prevention of post-operative adhesions in hamsters. Obstet Gynecol 78:858-60.

Coddington GC, Collins RL, Shawker TH, Anderson R, Loriaux DL, Winkel CA (1986): Long-acting gonadotropin hormone-releasing hormone analog used to treat uteri. Fertil Steril 45:624-29.

Costantini S, Anserini P, Valenzana M, Remorgida V, Venturini PL, DeCecco L (1990): Luteinizing hormone-releasing hormone analog therapy of uterine fibroid: analysis of results obtained with buserelin administered intranasally and goserelin administered subcutaneously as a monthly depot. Eur J Obstet Gynecol Reprod Biol 37:63-9.

Das K, Penney LL, Critser JK (1990): Effects of passive motion and early vs. delayed ambulation on adhesion formation in rat uterine surgery. Int J Fertil 35:245-8

deZiegler D, Bessis R, Frydman R (1991): Vascular resistance of uterine arteries: Physiological effects of estradiol and progesterone. Fertil Steril 55:775-779.

Diamond MP, Daniell JF, Johns D, et al. (1990): Adhesion formation and reformation after operative laparoscopy: assessment at early second-look procedures. 1990 AFS Annual Meeting prize paper.

Dicker RC, Greenspan JR, Strauss LT, et al. (1982): Complications of abdominal and vaginal hysterectomy among women of reproductive age in the United States. Am J Obstet Gynecol 144:841-6.

Drollette CM, Badawy SZA (1992): Pathophysiology of pelvic adhesions. Modern trends in preventing infertility. J Reprod Med 37:107-22.

Dubuisson JB, Lecuru F, Foulot H, Mandelbrot L, Aubriot FX, Mouly M (1991): Myomectomy by laparoscopy: a preliminary report of 43 cases. Fertil Steril 56:827-30.

Dunn RC (1991): A longitudinal study of adhesion reformation and de novo adhesion formation after laparoscopic adhesiolysis. 47th Annual meeting of the American Fertility Society. Abstract 0-013, S6).

Fedele L, Vercellini P, Bianchi S, Brioschi D, Dorta M (1990): Treatment with GnRH agonists before myomectomy and the risk of short-term myoma recurrence. Br J Obstet Gynaecol 97:393-6.

Filicori M, Hall DA, Loughlin JS, Rivier J, Vale W, Crowley WF Jr. (1983): A conservative approach to the management of uterine leiomyoma: pituitary desensitization by a luteinizing hormone-releasing hormone analogue. Am J Obstet Gynecol 147:726-7.

Friedman AJ, Barbieri RL, Doubilet PM, Fine C, Schiff I (1988): A randomized, double-blind trial of a gonadotropin releasing- hormone agonist (leuprolide) with or without medroxyprogesterone acetate in the treatment of leiomyomata uteri. Fertil Steril 49:404-9.

Friedman AJ, Rein MS, Harrison-Atlas D, Garfield JM, Doubilet PM (1989a): A randomized, placebo-controlled, double-blind study evaluating leuprolide acetate depot treatment before myomectomy. Fertil Steril 52:728-33.

Friedman AJ, Benacerraf B, Harrison-Atlas D, Gleason R, Barbieri RL, Shiff I (1989b): A randomized, placebo-controlled, double-blind study evaluating the efficacy of leuprolide acetate depot in the treatment of uterine leiomyomata. Fertil Steril 51:251-6.

Friedman AJ (1989c): Treatment of leiomyomata uteri with short-term leuprolide followed by leuprolide plus estrogen-progestin hormone replacement therapy for 2 years: a pilot study. Fertil Steril 51:526-8.

Friedman AJ (1989d): Vaginal hemorrhage associated with degenerating submucous leiomyomata during leuprolide acetate treatment. Fertil Steril 52:152-4.

Friedman AJ, Lobel SM, Rein MS, Barbieri RL (1990). Efficacy and safety considerations in women with uterine leiomyomas treated with gonadotropin-releasing hormone agonists: the estrogen threshold hypothesis. Am J Obstet Gynecol 163:1114-9.

Friedman AJ, Hoffman DI, Comite F, Browneller RW, Miller JD (1991): Treatment of leiomyomata uteri with leuprolide acetate depot: a double-blind, placebo-controlled, multicenter study. The Leuprolide Study Group. Obstet Gynecol 77:720-5.

Gutmann JN, Thornton KL, Carcangiu ML (1991): Histopathology of uterine myomata: evaluation of leuprolide acetate (LA) treatment. 47th Annual Meeting American Fertility Society. Abstract 0-107, S46.

Haney AF, Doty E (1992): Murine peritoneal injury and de novo adhesion formation caused by oxidized-regenerated cellulose (Interceed [TC7]) but not expanded polytetrafluoroethylene (Gore- Tex Surgical Membrane). Fertil Steril 57:202-208.

Healy DL, Lawson SR, Abbott M, Barid DT, Fraser HM (1986): Toward removing uterine fibroids without surgery: subcutaneous infusion of a luteinizing hormone-releasing hormone agonist commencing in the luteal phase. J Clin Endocrinol Metab 63:619-25.

Heinonen PK, Aine R, Seppala E (1990): Peritoneal fluid leukotriene B4 and prostaglandin E_2 in acute salpingitis. Gynecol Obstet Invest 29:292- .

Henzl MR, Corson SL, Moghissi K, Buttram VC, Berquist C, Jacobsen C (1988): Administration of nasal nafarelin as compared with oral danazol for endometriosis. NEJM 318:485-9.

Homm RJ, Garza DE, Mathur S, Austin M, Baggett B, Williamson HO (1989): Immunological aspects of surgically induced experimental endometriosis: variation in response to therapy. Fertil Steril 52:132-139.

Interceed (TC7) Adhesion Barrier Study Group (1989). Prevention of postsurgical adhesions by Interceed (TC7), an absorbable adhesion barrier: a prospective randomized multicenter clinical study. Fertil Steril 51:933-8.

Koziol DE, Holland PV, Alling DW, et al. (1986): Antibody to hepatitis B core antigen as a paradoxical marker for non-A, non-B hepatitis agents in donated blood. Ann Intern Med 104:488-95.

Levine RL (1985): Economic impact of pelviscopic surgery. J Reprod Med 30:655-59.

Luciano AA, Maier DB, Koch EI, Nulsen JC, Whitman GF (1989): A comparative study of postoperative adhesions following laser surgery by laparoscopy versus laparotomy in the rabbit model. Obstet Gynecol 74:220-4

Lumsden MA, West C, Baird DT (1987): Goserelin therapy before surgery for uterine fibroids. Lancet 1:36-7.

Lundorff P, Hahlin M, Kallfelt B, Thorburn J, Lindblom B (1991): Adhesion formation after laparoscopic surgery in tubal pregnancy: a randomized trial versus laparotomy. Fertil Steril 55:911-15.

Maheux R, Guilloteau C, Lemay A, Bastide A, Fazekas ATA (1984): Regression of leiomyomata uteri following hypoestrogenism induced by repetitive luteinizing hormone-releasing hormone agonist treatment: preliminary report. Fertil Steril 42:644-6.

Malone LJ (1969): Myomectomy: recurrence after removal of solitary and multiple myomas. Obstet Gynecol 34:200-3.

Marugo M, Centonze M, Bernasconi D, Fazzuoli L, Berta S, Giordana G (1989): Estrogen and progesterone receptors in uterine leiomyomas. Acta Obstet Gynecol Scand 68:731-5.

Mathur S, Garza DE, Smith LF (1990): Endometrial autoantigens eliciting immunoglobulin (Ig)G, IgA, and IgM responses in endometriosis. Fertil Steril 54:56-63.

Matta WHM, Stabile I, Shaw RW, Campbell S (1988): Doppler assessment of uterine blood flow changes in patients with fibroids receiving the gonadotropin-releasing hormone agonist Buserelin. Fertil Steril 49:1083-85.

Nakamura Y, Yoshimura Y, Yameda H, Ubukata Y, Ando M, Suzuki M (1991): Treatment of uterine leiomyomata with a luteinizing hormone-releasing hormone agonist: the possibility of nonsurgical management in selected perimenopausal women. Fertil Steril 55:900-5.

National Center for Health Statistics. Hysterectomies in the United States 1965-84. U.S. Department of Health, Education, and Welfare. DHEW publication no. (PHS) 88-1753. (Vital and health statistics; series B; no. 92.

Nezhat C, Nezhat F, Silfen SL, Schaffer N, Evans D (1991): Laparoscopic myomectomy. Int J Fertil 36:275-80.

Operative Laparoscopy Study Group (1991): Postoperative adhesion development after operative laparoscopy and evaluation at early second-look procedures. Fertil Steril 55:700-4.

Pagidas K, Tulandi T (1992): Effects of Ringer's lactate, Interceed (TC7) and Gore-Tex Surgical Membrane on postsurgical adhesion formation. Fertil Steril 57:199-201.

Pasqualini JR, Cornier E, Grenier J, Vella C, Schatz B, Netter A (1990): Effect of decapeptyl, an agonistic analog of gonadotropin-releasing hormone on estrogens, estrogen sulfates, and progesterone receptors in leiomyoma and myometrium. Fertil Steril 6:1012-1.

Perez RJ (1991): Second-look laparoscopy adhesiolysis, the procedure of choice for preventing adhesion recurrences. J Reprod Med 36:700-702.

Peterson HB, Hulka JF, Phillips JM. American Association of Gynecologic Laparoscopists' 1988 membership survey on operative laparoscopy. J Reprod Med 35:587.

Rosenberg SM (1990): Can we achieve adhesion-free surgery: The Female Patient, September, 4-8.

Rosenfeld DL (1986): Abdominal myomectomy for otherwise unexplained infertility. Fertil Steril 46:328-30.

Shaw RW (1989): Mechanism of LHRH analogue action in uterine fibroids. Horm Res 32:150.

Smith DC, Uhlir JK (1990): Myomectomy as a reproductive procedure. Am J Obstet Gynecol 162:1476-82.

Tamaya T, Fujimoto J, Okada H (1985): Comparison of cellular levels of steroid receptors in uterine leiomyoma and myometrium. Acta Gynecol Scand 64:307-9.

Thompson JN, Paterson-Brown S, Harbourne T, et al. (1989): Reduced human peritoneal plasminogen activating activity: Possible mechanism of adhesion formation. Br J Surg 76:382- .

Thorp JM, Jr., Katz VL (1991): Submucous myomas treated with gonadotropin releasing hormone agonist and resulting in vaginal hemorrhage. J Reprod Med 36:625-6.

Tulandi T, Collins JA, Burrows E, Jarrell JF, McInnes RA, Wrixon W, Simpson CW (1990): Treatment-dependent and treatment-independent pregnancy among women with periadnexal adhesions. Am J Obstet Gynecol 162:354-7.

Vietz P (1989): The value of pelviscopic myomectomy. Contemp Obstet Gynecol 105-9.

Vipond MN, Whawell SA, Thompson JN, et al. (1990): Peritoneal fibrinolytic activity and intra-abdominal adhesions. Lancet 335:1120.

Word RA, Odom MJ, Byrd W, Carr B (1990): The effect of gonadotropin-releasing hormone agonists on growth hormone secretion in adult premenopausal women. Fertil Steril 54:73-8.

Ylikorkala O: Treatment of uterine fibroids with nafarelin: results from the Finnish multicenter trial. Role of Nafarelin in Reproductive Medicine: A Worldwide Perspective. Presented at Washington, D.C., October 14, 1990.

Gynecologic Surgery and Adhesion Prevention, pages 187–190

ASHERMAN'S SYNDROME

Robert S. Neuwirth, M.D.
Director of Hysteroscopic Surgery
Babcock Professor of Obstetrics & Gynecology
College of Physicians and Surgeons of Columbia University
St. Luke's—Roosevelt Hospital Center
New York, NY 10025

ABSTRACT

Asherman's Syndrome was described by Asherman in 1948 as Amenorrhea Traumatica. Since the introduction of hysteroscopic surgery about 1970, an enlarging experience with the repair as well as the induction of intrauterine adhesions has been collected. The pathology and histologic processes involved in surgical repair and induction of scar in the uterus are discussed. The influence of the hormonal milieu as well as the special nature of endometrial repair as observed from the histologic evolution of the endometrium in menstruation are thought to be important factors in the induction and correction of intrauterine scar. While probably a special case, the endometrial model for healing appears to be fundamentally the same as other tissues.

ASHERMAN'S SYNDROME

In this Conference on Gynecological Surgery and Prevention of Adhesions, this is the only presentation about the prevention of adhesions in a space lined by an active epithelium. The fact that the tissue lining the space is an active epithelium and, indeed is hormonally influenced, is important to this discussion. It is possible to eradicate scar from the endometrial cavity so well that it is difficult if not impossible at times to identify grossly or microscopically where the scar had been. Such remarkable results appear to be the results of the nature of the repair process in the endometrium as well as the ability to manipulate it.

Asherman's syndrome was first described in 1948 as Amenorrhea traumatica.[1] It was seen in infertile and amenorrheic women who were found to have filling defects on hysterography. At hysterography, these filling defects may vary from filmy adhesions to thick scar.[2] Microscopically the adhesions may be fibrinous bands, avascular connective tissue, or vascularized scar. Islands of normal endometrium may be seen. Ninety per cent of the patients will give a history of post partum or post abortal hemorrhage requiring curettage and often a uterine infection co-exits. Therefore, the prime elements in most of the cases is a hypoestrogenic state, mechanical trauma (curettage), and probable concomitant clinical or subclinical infection. About 10 per cent of cases give no such history. Another group of patients where intrauterine adhesions can be seen is in postmenopausal women, presumably due to the prolonged hypoestrogenic state and possibly mild local inflammatory reaction to infection ascending from the vagina.

During the past fifteen years, an enlarging experience has been collected with the surgical induction of intrauterine scar performed under hysteroscopic control using laser coagulation[3] and electrosurgical resection and/or coagulation.[4] Curettage has sometimes been added to supplement the thermal injuries with mechanical abrasion. This work clearly shows that induction of scar can be achieved resulting in reduction or cessation of menstrual flow. The uterine cavity in these patients looks like the cases of intrauterine adhesion seen the Asherman's cases generally of the more severe variety. The most successful cases show not only adhesions of the epithelium but also myofibrous scars and even a cicatrix of the entire cavity leading to virtual obliteration of the space. The cavity which remains often is lined by a simple cuboidal epithelium beneath which is the myometrium. Islands of normal mucosa may be seen. This picture is reminiscent of the end result of a third degree burn of the skin.

It is possible to manipulate the outcomes of surgical repair of Asherman's syndrome as well as surgically induced endometrial scar. This experience sheds some light on the process of scar formation as well as epithelial repair in the endometrial cavity. There is no large clinicio-pathologic series of cases in which induction of endometrial scar by thermal injury through laser or electrosurgical burn has been done. However random cases are available. Reports of rates of amenorrhea following ablation are of some help but unfortunately we know that there is only a general correlation between the degree of scar and amenorrhea. The best clinical data on the hormonal impact on scar formation of which I am aware is Goldrath's report[5] on an increased frequency of amenorrhea following laser endometrial ablation if the patient was pretreated with Danazol. Our clinical experience with endometrial suppression before and following ablation also suggests enhanced scar formation in the hypoestrogenic state induced with gonadotropin agonists. If this is indeed true, it supports the hypothesis that the epithelial repair originates in islands of basalis glands which may start a repair process but in the presence of a hypoestrogenic state results in less epithelial regeneration than if normal or elevated estrogen levels circulate to the vessels supplying the uterus.

While not all centers use estrogen postoperatively in the repair of intrauterine scar, most do and I am not aware of any group who suppresses ovarian function following repair of Asherman's Syndrome. The presence of estrogen in the postoperative period is probably important in stimulating the residual endometrium which resurfaces the area where scar has been transected. Restoration of normal menses is high, about 90%, and indeed restoration of fertility occurs in about 50% of cases suggesting effective restoration of endometrium. Splinting the endometrium cavity with an IUD or balloon in the postoperative period is controversial.

The evolution of repair of the endometrium during normal menstrual shedding, has been studied by Ferenczy.[6] He has shown a resurfacing of the stroma in 24 hours by the basalis epithelium. There are no studies to evaluate the effect of the presence or absence of estrogen on this process, but it is known that on the first day of menstruation, plasma estrogen is relatively low. Ferenczy believes that the initial process of cell migration is estrogen independent but shortly thereafter these migrating cells multiply and the epithelium thickens under estrogen stimulation. Repair following diagnostic gynecologic curettage is evidently similar to the process following menstruation as it is rare to see intrauterine scar following only a diagnostic curettage. It is far more common following incomplete abortion and pregnancy termination and postpartum curettage when infection and a hypoestrogenic state are more likely and more prolonged than during the menstrual cycle.

Certainly the induction of and repair of scar of the endometrial epithelium is different than that seen on mesothelial surfaces. Peacock[7] reports that the denuded peritoneum will resurface with mesothelial cells in three to five days. There is poor hormonal sensitivity of the mesothelium of the peritoneal serosa although in pregnancy decidual nodules can sometimes be seen at cesarean section. The very rapid resurfacing of the endometrium following menstruation may not be fully analogous to the repair of the peritoneum as one insult is a specialized avascular necrosis of the superficial layers of the endometrium while the other is a response to an applied injury. However the difference in response to injury of peritoneal serosa and endometrium may be real as it is known that epithelium differs in various areas of the body and is under the influence of the underlying mesenchyme. This point is illustrated by the transformation of split thickness grafts of skin to the vaginal tube in reconstructive surgery in which the graft behaves as vaginal mucosa. Last, but not least, the endometrial epithelium is sensitive to estrogens, prostogens and androgens. What is not clear is when estrogen in particular begins to influence the endometrial epithelium in the repair process. Ferenczy describes the initial migration of the basalis cells without mitosis. He does not know if the migration is estrogen dependent but endometrial growth is. But even if migration is not estrogen sensitive the migration process is relatively rapid in the endometrium compared to the speed of fibroblast growth into fibrinous bands. Probably the rapid migration as well as the speed of early endometrial proliferation both help to protect the menstruating endometrium from forming adhesive bands. It also helps to explain the typical post-pregnancy curettage history related by ninety per cent of patients who present with documented Asherman's syndrome where the repair process may be retarded by infection, a hypoestrogenic state, and trauma.

Certainly the model presented by the endometrium is quite unique. It does not appear to differ fundamentally from the process of adhesion formation and epithelial repair in other areas of the body. But it does illustrate that there are differences in speed of the process in different organs and tissues, that hormonal modifications may play a role and that other factors are local and tissue specific: The search for interventions to modulate the repair/adhesion process toward specific therapeutic goals is young. The experience from Asherman's syndrome is instructive for improvement in the results of intrauterine surgery as well as for general consideration of the processes of scar induction and repair in other organs and tissues.

REFERENCES

1. Asherman JG: Amenorrhea Traumatica (Atretica). J Obstet Gynecol Br Emp 55:23-30, 1948.

2. Foix A, Bruno RO, Davison T, Baltasar L.: The pathology of postcurettage intrauterine adhesions. Am J Obstet Gynecol 96:1027-1033, 1966.

3. Goldrath MH, Fuller T, Segal S: Laser photovaporization of endometrium for the treatment of menorrhagia. Am J Obstet Gynecol 140:14-19, 1981.

4. Derman S, Rehnstrom J, Neuwirth RS: The long-term effectiveness of hysteroscopic treatment of menorrhagia and leiomyomas. Obstet Gynecol 77:591-594, 1991.

5. Goldrath MH: Use of Danazol in hysteroscopic surgery for menorrhagia. J Repro Med 35:91-96, 1990.

6. Ferenczy A, Bertrand G, Gelfand MM: Proliferation kinetics of human endometrium during the normal menstrual cycle. Am J Obstet Gynecol 133:859-867, 1979.

7. Peacock, E.: Wound Repair. Third Edition, W.B. Saunders Company, Philadelphia, PA, 1984.

Gynecologic Surgery and Adhesion Prevention, pages 191–204

PREVENTION OF POSTOPERATIVE ADHESIONS BY PRECOATING TISSUES WITH DILUTE SODIUM HYALURONATE SOLUTIONS

Eugene P. Goldberg
James W. Burns
Yoseph Yaacobi
Biomedical Engineering Center, Department of Materials Science & Engineering, University of Florida, Gainesville, FL 32611 (E.P.G., Y.Y)
Genzyme Corporation, Cambridge, MA 02139 (J.W.B.)

Postoperative adhesions (POA), the collagenous connective tissues which form in response to surgical trauma, can be a severe and life threatening surgical complication. However, no generally applicable methods are currently available to mitigate this often serious problem. We have investigated the use of dilute aqueous solutions of sodium hyaluronate (HA) as protective tissue coatings applied prior to surgical manipulation. In a random/blind rat cecal adhesions study conducted at three separate research centers, 0.4 wt% HA in buffered saline gave a three center average of 24% significant adhesions (n=74) versus 87% for phosphate buffered saline (PBS) controls (n=69). Histological data suggest that hyaluronic acid tissue precoating minimizes surgical trauma thereby inhibiting POA formation. Clinical studies have been initiated to evaluate the efficacy of tissue precoating with HA solutions in human surgery.

Most surgical procedures are accompanied by undesired tissue damage caused by cutting, desiccation, ischemia, and manipulative abrasion. Suture lines at closed incisions and anastomoses are known to be sites of adhesion formation as are areas of abrasive contacts that occur between tissue surfaces and the many instruments and devices used in surgery, i.e. sponges, gloves, aspirators, clamps, etc., which can severely damage cell membrane surfaces [1, 2]. We have previously shown that even momentary contact between fragile tissue membranes and hydrophobic plastic surfaces (e.g. between corneal endothelium and polymethylmethacrylate intraocular lens prostheses) can severely damage cell membranes [3]. The general wound-healing response to such tissue trauma can be the formation of unwanted collagenous connective tissue bridging adjacent damaged tissues or organs [4, 5]. These new internal connective tissues, postoperative adhesions (POA), which can form within one week following surgery [1], can be a serious complication following abdominal [6], thoracic [7], gynecologic [8], and orthopedic [9] surgery. For example, POA account for 80-90% of post-surgical intestinal obstructions, which occur following about 5% of all abdominal surgical procedures. They are the major cause of failure for infertility surgery. Adhesions place patients requiring cardiac reoperations at increased risk; resternotomy is associated with about a 5% incidence of major vascular injury with 35% mortality in patients experiencing major hemorrhage [10].

Other than microsurgical methods, previous research devoted to inhibiting adhesion formation has been directed at (a) mitigating the formation of fibrinous connective tissue [11], or (b) placing barriers between traumatized tissues at the conclusion of surgery after tissue damage has occurred; i.e. polymer solutions [12], Teflon films [13], or degradable oxidized regenerated cellulose (e.g. Interceed TC7 ™ [14]). These barrier methods may prove useful at specific sites of tissue injury such as at suture lines or deperitonealized surfaces. However, our approach to reducing POA formation has been to minimize the tissue damage caused by desiccation and handling during surgery by applying a protective tissue coating of an aqueous hydrophilic polymer solution immediately after entering the surgical field and before any significant surgical manipulation occurs. This protective polymer solution precoating must be biocompatible, not interfere with normal healing of incisions, and clear from the surgical site.

Our tissue precoating concept was investigated previously with solutions of low molecular weight polyvinylpyrrolidone (PVP) and dextran [4]. Although results with these materials provided encouraging POA reduction, the very high polymer concentrations required (20-40%), their poor handling properties in surgery, and questions concerning their biocompatibility, made these solutions clinically impractical. The principle objective of the research reported here, therefore,was to investigate the efficacy of low concentrations (<1.0%) of sodium hyaluronate (HA), the sodium salt of the natural polymer hyaluronic acid, for inhibiting adhesion formation.

Hyaluronic acid (HA) is a naturally occurring biocompatible high molecular weight mucopolysaccharide found in soft tissue and is a major component of the

Table 1: Effect of Tissue Precoating vs. Postcoating on Adhesion Formation in the Rat Cecal Abrasion Model

Group	Procedure	n/Group	Cecal Adhesions Total	%	≥2	%	Mean Total Score
1	A-RL	10	8	80	8	80	2.50
2	A-HA(0.6%)	10	9	90	8	80	3.50
3	HA(0.6%)-A-RL	10	1	10	1	10	0.20

Animals in the A-RL and A-HA (A-SOL) groups received no coating before abrasion, and received 6 ml test solution after abrasion. The HA-A-RL (SOL-A-RL) group received 5 ml HA solution coating before abrasion, 5 ml RL after abrasion. Cecal adhesions were scored one week after initial surgery according to the grading scale described in ref. 16.

extracellular matrix and synovial fluid [15]. The basic repeating unit of this polyelectrolyte polysaccharide is an alternating N-acetyl-glucosamine and D-glucuronic acid structure joined by β-1,3-glucuronidic and β-1,4-glucosaminidic bonds. Physiological solutions of HA exhibit non-Newtonian pseudoplastic rheological behavior, do not adversely affect wound healing, and are well suited for surgical use. We report here the results of a study to test the hypothesis that HA solutions might function effectively as tissue-protective coatings to reduce adhesion formation if administered before and during to surgical manipulations.
Preliminary studies employed a rat cecal abrasion model involving the application of HA solutions of various concentrations to the ceca of rats, prior to and after cecal abrasion (solution-abrasion-solution or SOL-A-SOL protocol). This resulted in a consistent reduction in the formation of cecal adhesions of grade 2 or higher as well as lower mean total scores of adhesions [16]. Since these studies were conducted employing the SOL-A-SOL protocol, further studies were carried out to delineate the relative effect on adhesion formation of tissue preprecoating vs. coating with HA solutions after abrasive trauma.

Data for these experiments are summarized in Table 1. Both 0.6% HA and Ringer's lactate (RL) groups yielded 80% grade 2 or higher POA when solutions were administered after abrasive trauma (A-SOL). However, tissue coating with 0.6% HA before abrasion followed by RL after abrasion (SOL-A-RL) gave only 10% grade 2 or higher POA. These results with SOL-A-RL are comparable to the SOL-A-SOL results for HA solutions. Additionally, the total incidence of cecal adhesions and the total mean score were also significantly lower in the test group that received the 0.6% HA solution prior to abrasion as compared to tissue coating with HA solution after the abrasion. These results suggested that (a) HA solutions afforded a marked degree of POA protection when applied to tissues before exposure to an abrasive manipulative insult, and (b) the HA solutions elicit their beneficial effect primarily by a mechanical rather than biochemical mechanism since the HA solution applied to the cecum and the abdominal cavity following abrasion had no observable effect on adhesion formation.

A much more extensive and statistically meaningful evaluation of the hypothesis that precoating with HA solutions could limit POA formation was conducted at three independent research centers employing the rat cecal abrasion model with some

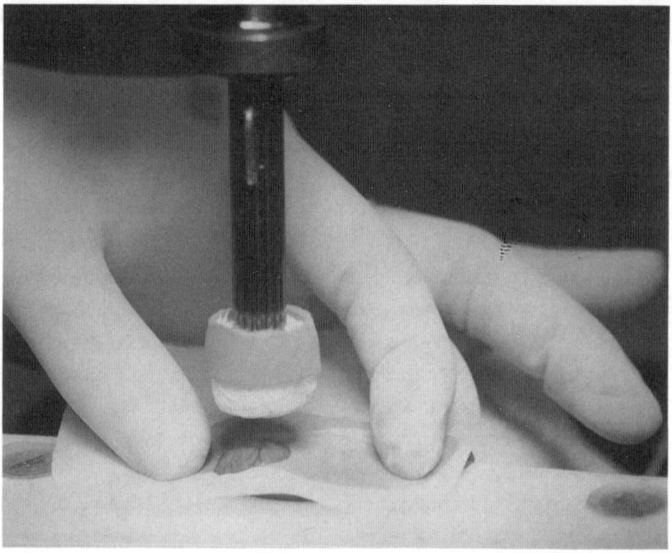

Fig. 1 Constant force, fixed area, rotary gauze abrasion apparatus shown in use with cecal holder.

Table 2: Averaged Multicenter Data

Group	% POA ≥ 2	n ≥ 2/Total n in Group
No Solution	72	52/72
PBS	87	60/69
0.1% HA	47	35/75
0.25% HA	40	30/74
0.4% HA	24	18/74

% animals with cecal adhesion scores of ≥ 2 using SOL-A procedure with autoabrader improvements in the protocol and abrasion procedure. The manual abrasion method used in our initial studies was similar to techniques reported before in the literature [5, 13]. However, some variability in the force and abrasion area can occur between animals and between different investigators performing the manual abrasion procedure. Thus, there are questions regarding reproducibility and the potential for inconsistent results using simple manual abrasion protocols. Therefore, to limit variability among the investigators at each independent site, and to minimize handling of the cecum by the abrader, we developed an instrument ("autoabrader") designed to more precisely control abrasion of the cecum.

After considering numerous prototypes, we selected a rotary autoabrader design. The device utilizes a rotating spline shaft which is free to move vertically. The constant abrasion force is controlled by the weight of the shaft so that small hand

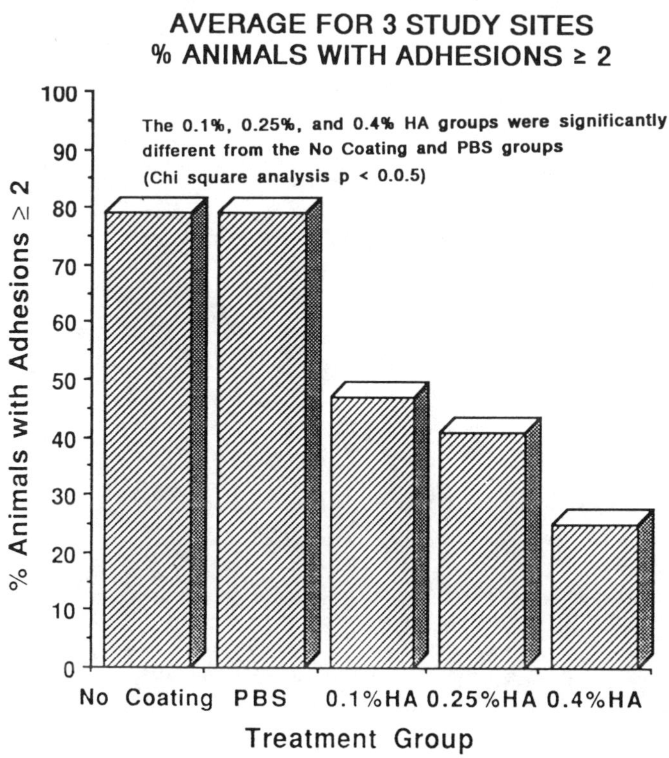

Fig 2. Summary of multicenter data for % significant adhesions vs. test solutions.

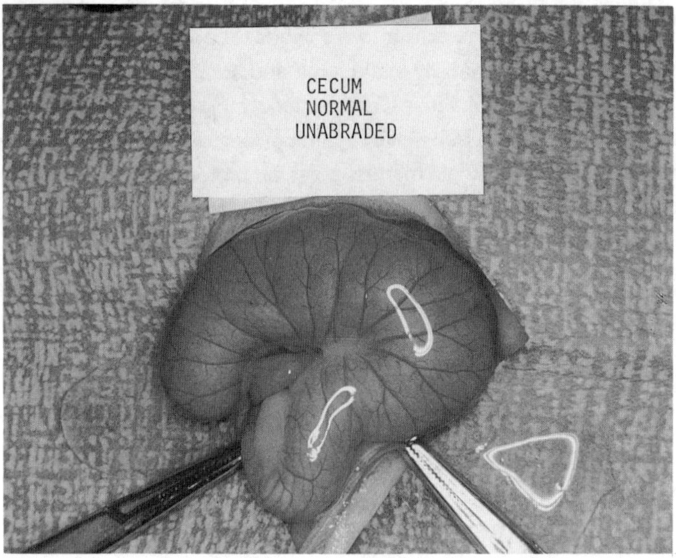
CECUM
NORMAL
UNABRADED

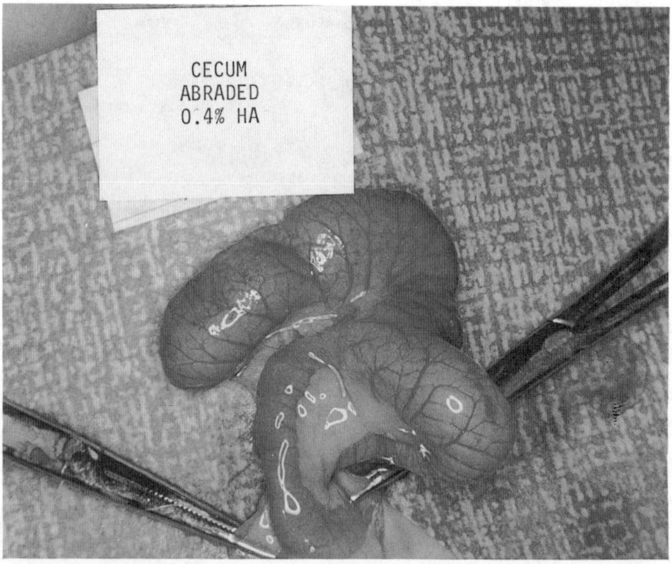
CECUM
ABRADED
0.4% HA

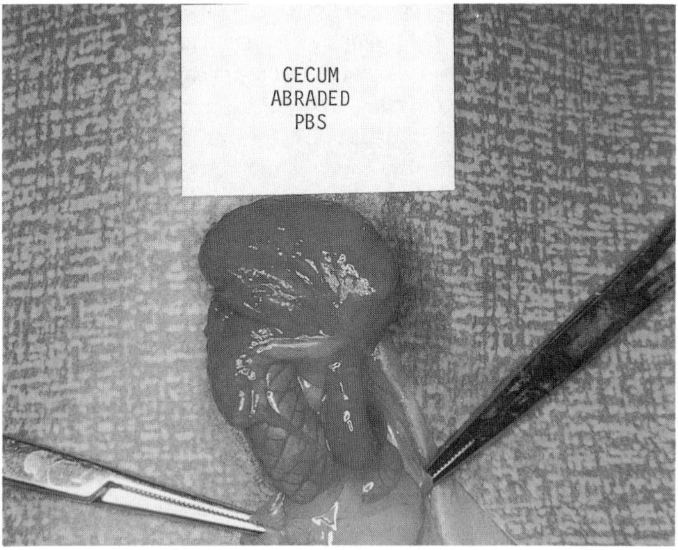

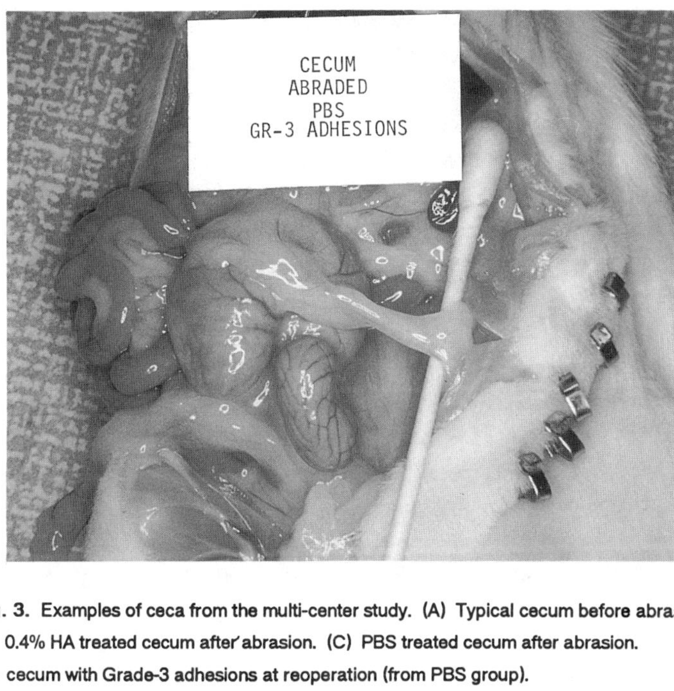

Fig. 3. Examples of ceca from the multi-center study. (A) Typical cecum before abrasion. (B) 0.4% HA treated cecum after abrasion. (C) PBS treated cecum after abrasion. (D) cecum with Grade-3 adhesions at reoperation (from PBS group).

movements will not change the abrading force. The shaft is connected to a battery-driven motor which controls shaft rotation at a constant rate. A counter mechanism records the number of shaft revolutions (abrasion cycles) and abrasion speed can be adjusted by a variable speed controller. The abrading surface used in all experiments was Type VII surgical gauze (1.77cm^2 surface area) secured to the end of the shaft by a rubber septum. The cecum was held during abrasion in a Teflon holding device which isolated the area of the cecum being abraded and prevented movement of the cecum during abrasion. The abrasion head spline shaft, and cecal holding device are shown in use in Figure 1.

Preliminary studies with the autoabrader and the surgical protocol defined tissue abrasion conditions required to consistently induce significant cecal adhesions (grade 2 or better) in 70%-90% of animals tested [17]. Parameters that were evaluated included, (1) abrasion force, (2) number of abrasion cycles, and (3) number of abrasion sites. The following conditions were used to induce a consistent level of adhesions: (1) 70 gm abrasion force, (2) 60 abrasion cycles per abrasion site, i.e. abrasion surface revolutions, (3) four cecal abrasion sites, and (4) 1.77 cm2 gauze surface area. These autoabrader conditions were used at all three research sites involved in the multicenter study. Test solutions were only applied prior to cecal abrasion (SOL-A precoating protocol) since the experiments summarized in Table 1 demonstrated that administration of HA solutions at the end of surgery had no effect on reducing adhesions.

Multicenter data are summarized in Table 2 and depicted graphically in Figure 2. Chi square analysis showed a statistically significant reduction in POA of Grade 2 and greater for all HA solutions. The largest POA inhibitory effect was observed for the 0.4% HA test group suggesting a concentration dependent response in the range 0.1 to 0.4% HA.

Reduced cecal damage for the HA treatment groups in the 3-center study was also clearly observed immediately following abrasion (Fig. 3A-D). The 0.4% HA treated ceca (Fig. 3B) exhibited less visible trauma and bleeding than the PBS treated ceca (Fig. 3C) indicative of the protective effect of the HA solution. A typical cecum from the PBS group showing Grade-3 adhesions at reoperation is shown in Figure 3D.

These results, from three separate laboratories, confirm that application of HA solutions prior to abrasive tissue trauma results in a statistically significant reduction in POA formation in the rat cecal adhesion model. The multicenter data strongly support our previous cecal POA data and convincingly indicate that HA solution precoating of tissues can be efficacious in reducing surgical tissue damage and consequent POA formation.

In a recent clinically relevant study using a canine pericardial abrasion model, we have also shown that tissue precoating with HA solutions affected a significant reduction in the incidence and severity of pericardial adhesions [18]. We therefore believe that tissue protective solutions of biocompatible, hydrophilic polymers, such as hyaluronic acid, can prove to be clinically useful in a wide variety of procedures, i.e. in gynecologic, abdominal, orthopedic, and cardio-thoracic surgery.

Histological evidence that tissue precoating with HA solutions provides protection from manipulative damage was obtained by staining and sectioning cecal tissue two days following abrasion performed according to the procedure used in the multicenter study [17]. By waiting two days after abrasion, the inflammatory response to the inflicted serosal trauma could be observed more readily than would be possible immediately following abrasion. In this experiment (Fig. 4A-C), the serosa of rat ceca coated with PBS consistently exhibited more extensive mesothelial hyperplasia, infiltration of inflammatory cells, and fibrinous exudate 2 days after cecal abrasion compared with the cecal serosa of animals treated with 0.4 wt% HA solution. PBS treated ceca had histology scores of 2 or higher for 90% of ceca (9/10) compared to 30% (3/10) for 0.4 wt% HA. In view of our rat cecal adhesions results, the mesothelial injury observed histologically in the PBS group is evidently sufficient to induce POA formation. Since HA solutions reduce POA in this model, we conclude that the precoating of tissues with HA solutions reduces tissue damage to the extent that POA do not readily form.

The formation of surgical adhesions appears to be the culmination of a series of biochemical events intended to repair tissue surfaces that have been injured during surgery. Studies on the etiology of POA formation [1, 2] indicate that rough handling, heavy gauze swabbing, surgical denudation, ischemia, cutting, and retraction cause tissue trauma and consequent adhesion formation. Almost immediately after surgical trauma, the wound site becomes permeable to a serosanguinous exudate containing wound healing mediators. Typically, within hours after tissue injury, a fibrin clot scaffold forms. This is then lysed within a few days by fibrinolytic plasmin which forms in response to the release of tissue plasminogen activator at the wound site. However, if fibrinolytic enzyme activity is inadequate to substantially lyse the fibrin within about 3 days, the fibrin can act as a scaffold for collagen synthesized by infiltrating fibroblasts resulting in the formation of POA, i.e. collagen bridging adjacent tissue damage sites.

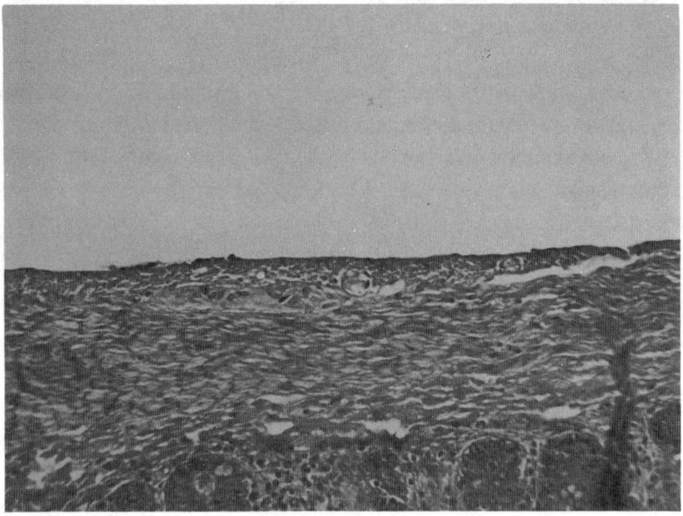

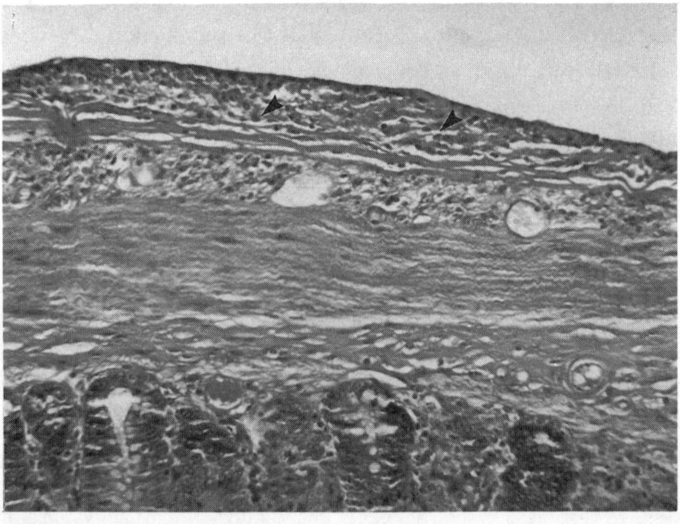

Fig. 4. Histology of rat cecal tissue: (4A) Normal unabraded cecum, (4B) cecum treated with 0.4% HA prior to abrasion showing only mild inflammatory response, and (4C) cecum treated with PBS before abrasion showing serosal damage, infiltration of inflammatory cells, and fibrinous exudate (arrows).

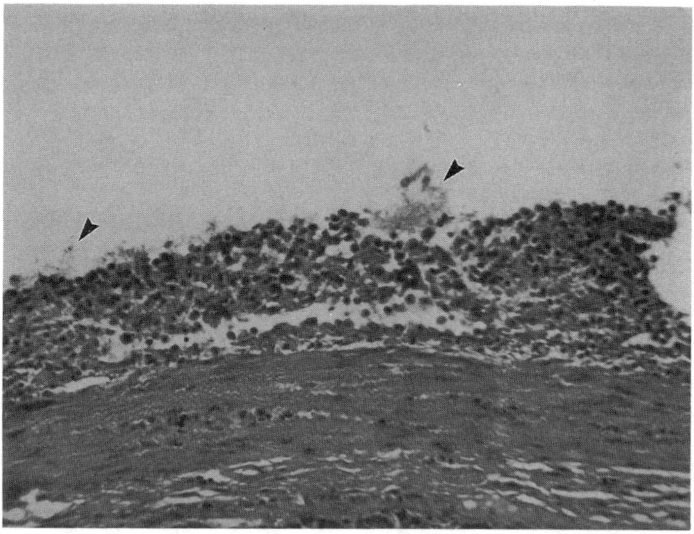

Raftery et al. [1] have shown that tissue abrasion and epithelial cell damage can decrease the release of plasminogen activator from injured tissue and thereby compromise the lysis of fibrin. This has also been observed following extensive surgical trauma caused by ischemia and desiccation as well as abrasion in cardiac and abdominal surgery [19]. An unlysed fibrin scaffold can therefore act as a matrix for infiltration of fibroblasts which produce the undesired collagenous connective tissue; i.e. the adhesions. We have shown histologically that HA solution coatings inhibit manipulative damage to tissue surfaces and thereby reduce the inflammatory processes which induce POA. It is therefore reasonable to expect less attenuation of plasminogen activation in tissues protected by HA solutions during surgery as compared to unprotected tissues. Fibrin would therefore be lysed normally and adhesions would be less likely to form.

The studies reported here suggest that solutions of biocompatible polymers may prove to be valuable adjuncts to surgical procedures as protective tissue coatings; coatings which can prevent severe manipulative trauma and thereby reduce the incidence and severity of POA. We conclude that HA, an important glycosaminoglycan which is found naturally in mammalian tissues, is particularly well suited for such tissue-protective solutions. We seek to confirm these observations in human clinical studies which are in progress.

References and Notes

1. H. Ellis, *Brit. J. Surg.*, **50**, 10 (1963); A. J. Raftery, *Eur. Surg. Res.*, **13**, 397 (1981).
2. G. B. Ryan, J. Grobety, G. Majno, *Ann. J. Pathol.*, **65**, 117 (1971); R. F. Buckman, P. D. Buckman, H. U. Hufnagel, R. Caldwell, *J. Surg. Res.*, **21**, 67 (1976); H. Ellis, *World J. Surg.*, **4**, 303 (1980); G. Holtz, *Fertil. Steril.*, **41**, 497 (1984); J. J. Stangel, J. D. Nisbet, H. Settles, *J. Reprod. Med.*, **29**, 143 (1984).
3. H. E. Kaufman, J. Katz, J. Valenti, J. W. Sheets, E. P. Goldberg, *Science*, **198**, 525 (1977).
4. E. P. Goldberg, J. W. Sheets, M. B. Habal, *Arch. Surg.*, **115**, 776 (1980).
5. D. A. Duncan, Y. Yaacobi, E. P. Goldberg, M. Mines, M. J. Carmichael, *J. Surg. Res.*, **45**, 44 (1988).
6. W. F. Becker, *Surg. Gynec. Obstet.*, **95**, 472 (1952); P. Nemir, *Ann. Surg.*, **135**, 367 (1952); J. F. Perry, G. A. Smith, E. G. Yonehiro, *Ann. Surg.*, **142**, 810 (1955); L. E. Raf, Acta Chir. Scand., **135**, 67 (1969).
7. W. J. Cliff, J. Grobetz, G. B. Ryan, *J. Thorac. Cardiovasc. Surg.*, **54**, 744 (1973); W. J. Cliff, G. B. Ryan, *ibid.*, **65**, 744 (1973); J. Gallo, E. Artinano, C. G. Duran, *ibid.*, **89**, 709 (1985); R. DePaulis et al., *J. Cardiovasc. Surg.*, **31**, 202 (1990).
8. V. Gomel, *Fertil Steril.*, **40**, 607 (1983); V. Gomel, *Curr. Probl. Obstet. Gynecol.*, **1**, 10 (1978); C. A. Eddy, R. H. Asch, J. P. Balmaceda, *Fertil. Steril.*, **33**, 557 (1980).
9. S. A. Meyers, A. V. Seaber, R. R. Glisson, J. A. Nunley, *J. Orthopaedic Res.*, **7**, 683 (1989); S. C. Thomas, L. C. Jones, D. S. Hungerford, *Clin. Orthopaedics Rel. Res.*, **206**, 281 (1986); A. D. Potenza, *J. Bone Jt. Surg.*, **45A**, 1217 (1963).
10. R. C. Dobell and A. K. Iain, *Ann. Thorac. Surg.*, **37**, 273 (1984); F. D. Loop, *ibid.*, **37**, 271 (1984).
11 G. Holtz, *J. Reprod. Res.*, **24**, 141 (1980).
12. M. R. Soules, L. Dennis, A. Bosarge, D. E. More, *Am. J. Obstet. Gynecol.*, **143**, 829 (1982); T. Elkins, R. Bury, J. Ritter, F. Ling, R. Ahokas, C. Homsey, L Malinak, *Fertil. Steril.*, **41**, 926 (1984); C. M. Fredericks, et al., *Am. J. Obstet. Gynecol.*, **155**, 667 (1986); M. P. Diamond, et al., *Intn. J. Fertil.*, **33**, 278 (1988).
13. S. P. Boyers, M. P. Diamond, A. H. DeCherney, *Fertil. Steril.*, **49**, 1066 (1988).
14. Interceed (TC7) Adhesion Barrier Study Group, *Fertil. Steril.*, **51**, 933 (1989); T. Shimanuki, K. Nishimura, F. Montz, R. Nakamura, G. diZerega, *J. Biomed. Mtls. Res.*, **21**, 173 (1987).
15. W. D. Comper and T. C. Laurent, *Physiol. Rev.*, **58**, 255 (1978); C. Weiss and E. A. Balasz, in *Mediguide to Orthopedics*, **Vol. 4**, 1, eds. W. L. Jaffee and M. G. Neuwirth, Carter-Wallace, Cranbury, NJ (1984).
16. In preliminary experiments different concentrations of HA formulated in two solution media, buffered saline (PBS) and Ringer's lactate (RL), were studied in a rat cecal abrasion model. Results of these experiments are summarized below:

Data from Initial Studies on the Effect of Tissue Precoating with HA Solutions (in 2 aqueous Media) on POA in a Rat Cecal Abrasion Model (SOL-A-SOL procedure). Complete data to be published.

Solution	Aqueoul Medium	n/Group	Cecal Adhesions ≥2	Cecal Adhesions %	Mean Total Score
RL (control)	RL	25	15	60	2.4
0.1% HA	RL	10	0	0	0.4
0.3% HA	RL	18	3	17	0.9
0.6% HA	RL	19	0	0	0.0
0.1% HA	PBS	10	2	20	0.9
0.6% HA	PBS	10	0	0	0.2

HA was used as a highly purified sodium salt. The surgical protocol involved a mid-line dorsal incision and controlled gauze (Type VII surgical gauze) abrasion (20 strokes) of the dorsal and ventral cecal surfaces with various modes of test solution application. Abdominal tissues of each animal (200-300 gm Sprague-Dawley female rats) were coated with 6 ml of solution before abrasion and 6 ml after abrasion before closure of the incision; i.e. SOL-A-SOL. Adhesions were scored at 7-14 days after the initial surgery according to the following numerical grading system: 0 - No Adhesions,1 - Filmy Adhesions/Easily Dissected Plane, 2 - Mild Adhesions/Dissectable Plane, 3 - Moderate Adhesions/Difficult Dissection, and 4 - Dense Adhesions/Nondissectable. The percent "significant adhesions" (scored as grade 2 or higher) was used as a convenient and statistically meaningful means of comparative evaluation. Data are also given for "Mean Total Scores", the total of all adhesion scores per group divided by the total number of animals/group.

17. The following general protocol was used for the multi-center study: (a) the cecum was coated before abrasion with 4 ml of test solution (b) the round abrading surface had an area of 1.8 cm^2 of type VII surgical gauze, (c) the cecum was secured during abrasion in a Teflon holder that contained a hole large enough to accommodate the rotating abrasion surface, (d) the abrasion load was 70 g, (e) each of four abrasion sites on the cecum received 60 complete revolutions (abrasion cycles) at 130 rpm, (f) female Sprague Dawley rats, 200-250 g, were used, (g) animals were anesthetized by i.m. injection of ketamine, 100 mg/kg, and xylazine, 10 mg/kg, (h) animals were sacrificed one week following the traumatic surgical procedure by CO_2 asphyxiation and graded for POA after a left paramedial incision through the skin and peritoneum, (i) all surgical procedures and POA grading were conducted random/blind, and (j) the groups studied were: A- No Coating, B- PBS, C- 0.1% HA in PBS, D- 0.25% HA in PBS, and E- 0.4% HA in PBS. Each test group consisted of approximately 25 rats. Detailed study to be published.
18. The following table summarizes data excerpted from a collaborative canine pericardial adhesions study with Drs. A. Kaelin, J.C. Bailey, E.D. Staples, and J.M. Seeger (Dept. Surgery, University of Florida Medical Center) to be published:

Effect of HA Solution Precoating on POA in a Canine Pericardial Adhesions Model (n=5/group)

Tissue Coating Solution	Right Pericardium (Unabraded)		Left Pericardium (Abraded)	
	≥2	Mean Total Score	≥2	Mean Total Score
RL	0%	0.4	60%	1.6
0.1% HA in RL	0%	0.0	0%	0.0
0.4 % HA in RL	0%	0.0	20%	0.6

This experiment compared RL, 0.1 wt% HA, and 0.4 wt% HA solutions in RL using 15 dogs; 5 dogs per solution. The protocol included: (1) a left thoracotomy at the fifth intercostal space, (2) all instruments, gauze sponges, and gloves dipped in study solution prior to surgical manipulations, (3) coating of external pericardial surface with 25 ml of test solution, (4) pericardiotomy followed by coating of the epicardium and inner surface of the pericardium (pericardial sac) with 25 ml test solution, (5) controlled gauze sponge abrasion of the left epicardium and inner surface of the pericardium, but no abrasion to the right side, (6) coating of the pericardial sac with 25 ml test solution, (7) exposure of the pericardial cavity to the air for 30 minutes to simulate surgical desiccation, (8) irrigation and suctioning of the pericardial sac with 25 ml RL solution to simulate surgical removal of clots and debris from the surgical field, (9) biopsy of the pericardium before the initial tissue coating and after desiccation; (10) coating of the pericardial cavity with 25 ml test solution prior to closing. Adhesions were scored random/blind according to the grading system in ref. 16 by 3 surgeons.

19. J. N. Thompson, et al., *Brit. J. Surg.*, **76**, 382 (1989); M. N. Vipond, S. A. Whawell, J. N. Thompson, H. A. F. Dudley, *Lancet*, **335**, 1120 (1990).

20. Management and surgery of all animals were in fully accredited facilities in accordance with the Federal Animal Welfare Act and the *NIH Guide for Care and Use of Laboratory Animals*.

21. We wish to thank Dr. Roderick Bronson, D.V.M., of the Department of Pathology, Tufts School of Veterinary Medicine, for evaluation of the rat cecal histology specimens.

22. One author (E. P. Goldberg) wishes to express his appreciation to Dr. Mutaz Habal for stimulating his interest in the problem of abdominal adhesion prevention.

23. Research support from the State of Florida Biomedical Engineering Center of Excellence and from the Genzyme Corp., Cambridge, MA is gratefully acknowledged.

Gynecologic Surgery and Adhesion Prevention, pages 205–212

IMPROVING THE EFFICACY OF INTERCEED BARRIER IN THE PRESENCE OF BLOOD USING THROMBIN, HEPARIN OR A BLOOD INSENSITIVE BARRIER, MODIFIED INTERCEED (nTC7)

D.M. Wiseman, L.F. Kamp, L. Saferstein,
C.B. Linsky, L.E. Gottlick, and M.P. Diamond
Ethicon, Inc., Somerville, New Jersey 08876 (DMW, LFK, CBL, LEG)
Noramco, Inc., New Brunswick, New Jersey 08903 (LS)
Department of Obstetrics and Gynecology, Vanderbilt University, Nashville, Tennessee 37232 (MPD)

INTRODUCTION

Meticulous hemostasis is always desirable for the prevention of adhesions (Buckman et al., 1976; Cliff et al., 1973; Ryan et al., 1971). However, while focal areas of bleeding may be controlled with cautery or ligature, it is sometimes difficult to control diffuse oozing from raw surfaces. In addition to increasing fibrin deposition *per se*, bleeding at a surgical site can compromise the ability of INTERCEED [(R)] (TC7) Absorbable Adhesion Barrier to reduce adhesion formation (Linsky et al., 1988). Therefore meticulous hemostasis must be achieved before application of INTERCEED Barrier (package insert, INTERCEED Barrier, ETHICON, Inc.).

Because meticulous hemostasis is not always achievable, we investigated how the blood sensitivity of INTERCEED Barrier may be overcome, using three approaches in animal models: use of thrombin, use of heparin and use of a modified INTERCEED Barrier.

A.USE OF THROMBIN TO CONTROL BLEEDING FROM DIFFUSE SITES

Although a number of methods exist for the control of bleeding, many of them (cautery, ligature) are more suited for the control of focal bleeders than for diffuse areas of capillary bleeding or "oozing". Thrombin and fibrin sealant are two agents which are more suited for control of "oozing" and which are employed in general or cardiovascular surgery (Kram et al., 1990; Spotnitz et al., 1987). These agents do not induce thermal damage. There is concern that these agents may enhance adhesion formation which has been reported in some animal studies (Gauwerky et al., 1990). However, in other studies, the application of thrombin does not worsen adhesions (McGaw et al., 1988), and the application of fibrin sealant actually reduced adhesion formation (Lindenberg et al., 1985; de Virgilio et al., 1990; Tulandi et al., 1992; Caballerro and Tulandi, 1992).

We have conducted studies to test the hypothesis that thrombin is a suitable agent for achieving hemostasis without exacerbating adhesions, and whether its use at sites of bleeding facilitates the efficacious use of INTERCEED Barrier in the prevention of adhesions (Wiseman et al., 1992). We also tested whether, after hemostasis with thrombin, the combination of INTERCEED Barrier and heparin still demonstrated improved efficacy over INTERCEED Barrier alone, as we have shown previously in animal studies (Diamond et al., 1991a,b).

To examine these issues, a standard abrasion of the rabbit uterine horn (Linsky et al., 1987) with two levels of bleeding superimposed (Wiseman et al., 1992) was utilized to represent the range of conditions which could be described as "diffuse capillary bleeding". At the lower end of the range (the "oozing" model), the punctate bleeding induced by scalpel blade abrasion of the rabbit uterus was allowed to continue in contrast to our standard model in which bleeding is controlled by tamponade. At the upper end of this range (the "bleeding" model) each of four blood vessels on each uterine ligament were nicked to produce a heavier degree of bleeding, which would normally require cautery or ligature for control. These two models were performed separately.

After creating the uterine horn lesions, the following treatments were randomly revealed to the surgeon:

1) Control - "Oozing" or "Bleeding" were allowed to stop spontaneously.
2) INTERCEED(R) (TC7) Absorbable Adhesion Barrier (ETHICON, Inc. Somerville, New Jersey) was wrapped around each bleeding uterine horn and moistened with saline.
3) Thrombin (1000 units/ml, Thrombin Topical USP Thrombogen, Johnson & Johnson Medical, Inc, Arlington, Texas) was used to achieve hemostasis. No effort was made to remove the clots which were substantial in the "bleeding" model. Two minutes were allowed to elapse before the uterine horns were returned to the abdomen.
4) Thrombin-induced hemostasis, application of INTERCEED Barrier and moistening with saline.
5) Thrombin-induced hemostasis followed by INTERCEED Barrier application and moistening with heparin (1000U/horn as per Diamond et al., 1991a).
6) Thrombin soaked into INTERCEED Barrier. In the "oozing" model only, INTERCEED Barrier was placed over the oozing site. Thrombin was then applied to the blood-soaked fabric.

In groups 3, 4 and 5, treatments were revealed in a staged fashion, that is the random assignment to an INTERCEED Barrier group was not revealed until hemostasis with thrombin was achieved.

Two weeks later, adhesions were assessed by measuring the length of adherent uterine horn (Figures 1 and 2) and by noting the number of uterine horns which were completely free of adhesions.

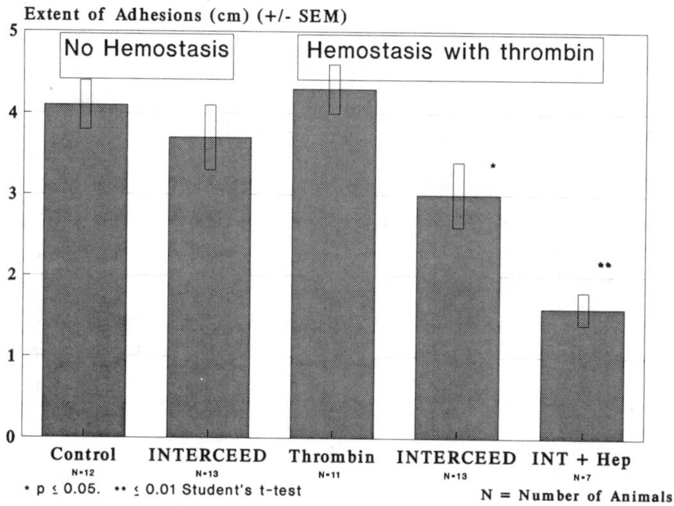

Figure 1. Effect of INTERCEED Barrier in the rabbit uterine horn "bleeding" model, with and without thrombin hemostasis.

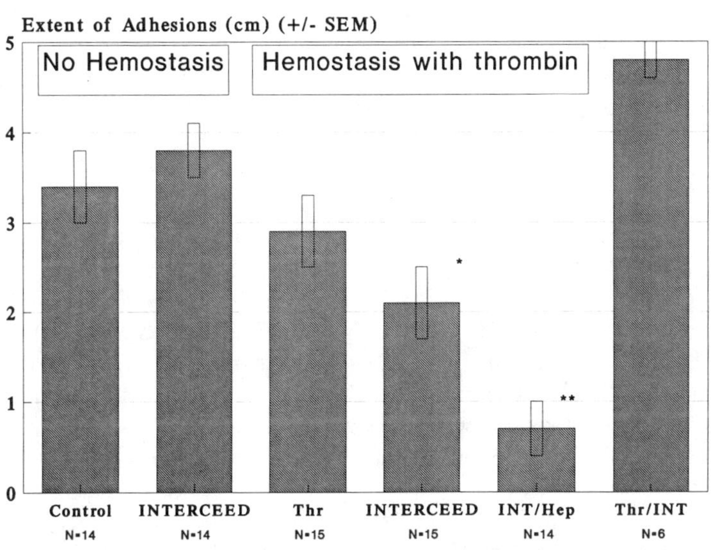

Figure 2. Effect of INTERCEED Barrier in the rabbit uterine horn "oozing" model, with and without thrombin hemostasis.

The following observations from both the bleeding and oozing models (Figures 1 and 2 respectively) were made:

1. The use of thrombin to achieve hemostasis in either the "bleeding" or "oozing" models did not worsen adhesion formation, compared with controls. In the "oozing" model thrombin reduced the extent of adhesions and increased the incidence of adhesion-free horns (4/30 vs 0/28, for controls) but these effects were not statistically significant.

   In contrast to previous studies (McGaw et al., 1988), the lack of a detrimental effect of thrombin may have been due to the hemostasis protocol. Clotting was allowed to proceed to completion for at least two minutes before returning organs to the abdomen. Replacement of organs during clotting may have enhanced fibrinous adhesions.
2. Application of INTERCEED Barrier to "bleeding" or "oozing" surfaces without achieving hemostasis, did not reduce adhesion formation, confirming previous observations (Linsky et al., 1988).
3. Application of INTERCEED Barrier to "bleeding" or "oozing" surfaces, after the achievement of hemostasis with thrombin, reduced adhesion formation. This significant effect occurred despite the presence of large clots in the "bleeding" model. Clinically however, effort should be made to reduce fibrin deposition wherever possible.
4. The beneficial effect of using thrombin on the efficacy of INTERCEED Barrier was not observed (in the "oozing" model) if thrombin was applied to blood-soaked INTERCEED Barrier. In fact, adhesions were more extensive under these conditions.
5. The efficacy of INTERCEED Barrier (applied after use of thrombin) in both models was further enhanced when moistened with heparin. In the "oozing" model, there were large numbers of horns (14/28) completely devoid of adhesions, compared with controls (0/28) ($p \leq 0.001$, Fisher's Exact test).

B. USE OF INTERCEED BARRIER PLUS HEPARIN AT A BLEEDING SITE

It has previously been shown in animals that heparin enhances the efficacy of INTERCEED Barrier in both adhesion formation (Diamond et al., 1991a) and adhesion reformation (Diamond et al., 1991b) models. In addition, heparin reverses the detrimental effect that blood has on the efficacy of INTERCEED Barrier (Linsky et al., 1988). In this study involving a standard rabbit uterine horn model, blood was allowed to soak into INTERCEED Barrier. Under these conditions, the barrier was no longer effective. When blood was placed on INTERCEED Barrier that was already soaked in heparin solution, efficacy was maintained (Diamond et al., 1988, Linsky et al., 1988).

In surgical practice, blood is not placed on INTERCEED Barrier, rather INTERCEED Barrier could be placed (inappropriately) at a site that is bleeding. Using the "bleeding" rabbit uterine horn model, we conducted a study in which

INTERCEED Barrier was placed on an actively bleeding and injured site, and moistened immediately with heparin solution (1000 units/ml/horn). The results (Table 1) show that INTERCEED Barrier plus heparin reduced adhesions when placed over actively bleeding and injured uterine horns.

Table 1: Efficacy of INTERCEED Barrier Plus Heparin in a "Bleeding" Uterine Horn Model With No Hemostasis

Treatment	N animals	Extent [a] (cm) + SEM	% Free [c] horns
Control	6	3.3 ± 0.81	8
INTERCEED + heparin	7	1.3 ± 0.48 [b]	43

[a] = Extent of adhesions (cm) per uterine horn
[b] = $p \leq 0.05$ vs Control (Student's t-test)
[c] = Percentage of all horns studied with complete absence of adhesions ($p \leq 0.01$, Fisher's Exact test)

There are several explanations for this positive effect of heparin. Mechanistically, heparin might hinder fibrin deposition (and enhance its removal) on the surface and within the interstices of the INTERCEED Barrier fabric, preventing the inclusion of the fabric in a fibrinous adhesion.

C. USE OF MODIFIED INTERCEED (nTC7), AN ABSORBABLE ADHESION BARRIER WITH RELATIVE INSENSITIVITY TO BLOOD

We have discovered (Saferstein et al., 1992) that a modified form of INTERCEED Barrier (nTC7) has some unique properties. We have evaluated its use for the prevention of adhesions in three animal models.

Use of nTC7 at Sites of Good Hemostasis

The effects of INTERCEED Barrier, INTERCEED Barrier plus heparin and nTC7 were compared using the rabbit uterine horn abrasion model (Linsky et al., 1987). The results in Table 2 show that nTC7 was more efficacious than INTERCEED Barrier and functions as well as the combination of INTERCEED Barrier plus heparin.

Use of nTC7 in a Model of Adhesion Reformation

The similarity between nTC7 and INTERCEED Barrier plus heparin was further evaluated in an adhesion reformation model in the rabbit. Two weeks after a standard uterine horn abrasion, adhesiolysis was performed as described by Diamond et al.

Table 2: Efficacy of Modified INTERCEED Barrier (nTC7) in a "Standard" Uterine Horn Model (With Meticulous Hemostasis)

Treatment	N animals	Extent [a] (cm) + SEM	% Free [b] horns
Control	13	3.2 ± 0.42	8
INTERCEED Barrier	13	1.5 ± 0.42 [c]	15
nTC7	12	0.4 ± 0.15 [c]	58 [d]
INTERCEED + heparin	7	0.3 ± 0.13 [c]	71 [d]

[a] = Extent of adhesions (cm) per uterine horn
[b] = Percentage of all horns with no adhesions
[c] = $p \leq 0.01$ vs Control (Student's t test)
[d] = $p \leq 0.01$ vs Control or INTERCEED (Fisher's Exact test)

(1991b). Only animals with an extent of adhesions greater than 1 cm on each horn were entered into the study. Treatments were randomly applied as below. Two weeks later, the extent of adhesions was assessed by estimating the percent (%) of the total horn length with adhesions.

The formation of adhesions prior to adhesiolysis did not differ significantly among the animals entered into the three groups (data not shown). Both nTC7 and INTERCEED Barrier plus heparin significantly reduced the extent of adhesions (Table 3). However only in the group treated with INTERCEED Barrier plus heparin was the incidence of adhesions reduced significantly.

Table 3: Efficacy of Modified INTERCEED Barrier in a Reformation Uterine Horn Model of Adhesions

Treatment	N animals	Extent [a] (%) + SEM	% Free [b] horns
Control	7	88 ± 5	0
nTC7	7	29 ± 8 [c]	14
INTERCEED + Heparin	9	19 ± 8 [c]	33 [d]

[a] = Extent of adhesions (% of horn length) per uterine horn, per animal
[b] = Percentage of all horns studied with complete absence of adhesions
[c] = $p \leq 0.01$ vs Control (Student's t-test)
[d] = $p \leq 0.05$ vs Control (Fisher's Exact test)

Effect of nTC7 at Sites of Poor Hemostasis

Using the "bleeding" model described earlier we found that nTC7 reduced the extent and incidence of adhesions, while INTERCEED Barrier was not effective, as expected, (Saferstein et al., 1992; Table 4). The reduction in the incidence and extent of adhesions obtained with nTC7 was at least as good as that observed previously with INTERCEED Barrier plus heparin under similar conditions (see above).

Table 4: Efficacy of Modified INTERCEED Barrier in a "Bleeding" Uterine Horn Model With No Hemostasis

Treatment	N animals	Extent [a] (cm) + SEM	% Free [b] horns
Control	15	4.4 ± 0.19	0
INTERCEED Barrier	14	3.6 ± 0.40	7
nTC7	19	0.7 ± 0.15 [c]	45 [d]

[a] = Extent of adhesions (cm) per uterine horn
[b] = Percentage of all horns studied with no adhesions
[c] = $p \leq 0.01$ vs Control or INTERCEED (Student's t test)
[d] = $p \leq 0.01$ vs Control (Fisher's Exact test)

CONCLUSION

In an effort to improve upon the performance of INTERCEED Barrier, particularly at sites of poor hemostasis, we have made a number of observations in animals, from which the following conclusions may be drawn.

1. Use of thrombin for hemostasis at oozing sites does not enhance adhesion formation.
2. In effecting hemostasis, thrombin does not compromise the efficacy of INTERCEED Barrier.
3. Heparin added to INTERCEED Barrier improves the reduction in adhesion formation, with or without hemostasis. However, in the presence of blood, the absorption rate of the fabric is retarded.
4. A modified INTERCEED Barrier (nTC7), reduces adhesion formation, even when hemostasis is far from adequate, and without the necessity for heparin. Materials such as nTC7 which are relatively "blood insensitive" are likely to find a broader use in adhesion prevention than those which are not.

ACKNOWLEDGEMENT

It is a pleasure to acknowledge the technical support of Kathy Hiemer, Hitoshi Kanke and Deborah Daly, and the valuable comments of Timothy Cunningham, Timothy Kiorpes and Douglas Johns.

REFERENCES

Buckman RF, Woods M, Sargent L, Gervin AS (1976): A unifying pathogenetic mechanism in the etiology of intraperitoneal adhesions: J Surg Res 20:1-5.

Caballero J, Tulandi T (1992): Effects of Ringer's lactate and fibrin glue on postsurgical adhesions. J Reprod Med 37:141-143.

Cliff WJ, Groberty J, Ryan GB (1973): Postoperative pericardial adhesions. The role of mild serosal injury and spilled blood. J Thorac Cardiovasc Surg 65:744-750.

de Virgilio C, Dubrow T, Sheppard BB, MacDonald WD, Nelson RJ, Lesavoy MA, Robertson JM (1990): Fibrin glue inhibits intra-abdominal adhesion formation. Arch Surg 125:1378-1382.

Diamond MP, Linsky CB, Cunningham T, Kamp L, Wiseman D, diZerega G (1988): Effect of the combination of glycosaminoglycans with TC7 (INTERCEED)* in the reduction of adhesions. Fertil Steril (Prog Suppl) 51:S33-34.

Diamond MP, Linsky CB, Cunningham T, Kamp L, Pines E, DeCherney AH, diZerega GS (1991a): Synergistic effects of INTERCEED(TC7)* and heparin in reducing adhesion formation in the rabbit uterine horn model. Fertil Steril 55:389-394.

Diamond MP, Linsky CB, Cunningham T, Kamp L, Pines E, DeCherney AH, diZerega, GS (1991b): Adhesion reformation: reduction by the use of INTERCEED R (TC7) plus heparin. J Gyn Surg 7:1-6.

Gauwerky JFH, Mann J, Bastert G (1990): The effect of fibrin glue and peritoneal grafts in the prevention of intraperitoneal adhesions. Arch Gynecol Obstet 247:161-166.

Kram HB, Tirso J, Clark SR, Hermenegildo PO, Shoemaker WC (1990): Techniques of splenic preservation using fibrin glue. J Trauma 30:97-101.

Lindenberg S, Steentoft P, Sorensen SS, Olesen HP (1985): Studies on the prevention of intra-abdominal adhesion formation by fibrin sealant. Acta Chir Scand 151:525-527.

Linsky CB, Diamond MP, Cunningham T, Constantine, B, DeCherney AH, diZerega G (1987): Adhesion reduction in the rabbit uterine horn model using an absorbable barrier - TC7. J Reprod Med 32:17-20.

Linsky CB, Diamond MP, DeCherney AH, diZerega GS, Cunningham T (1988): Effect of blood on the efficacy of barrier adhesion reduction in the rabbit uterine horn model. Infertility 11:273-280.

McGaw T, Elkins TE, DeLancey JOL, McNeeley SG, Warren J (1988): Assessment of intraperitoneal adhesion formation in a rat model: can a procoagulant substance prevent adhesions? Obstet Gynecol 71:774-778.

Ryan GB, Groberty J, Majno G (1971): Postoperative peritoneal adhesions. A study of mechanisms. Am J Path 65:117-148.

Saferstein L, Wolf S, Kamp LK, Linsky CB, Wiseman D (1992): Process for preparing a neutralised oxidized cellulose product and its method of use. US Patent 5134229.

Spotnitz WD, Dalton MS, Baker JW, Nolan SP (1987): Reduction of perioperative hemorrhage by anterior mediastinal spray application of fibrin glue during cardiac operations. Ann Thor Surg 44:529-531.

Tulandi T (1991): Effects of fibrin sealant on tubal anastomosis and adhesion formation. Fertil Steril 56:136-138.

Wiseman DM, Gottlick LE, Diamond MP (1992). Hemostasis at a bleeding site using thrombin: Efficacy of INTERCEED (R) (TC7) Absorbable Adhesion Barrier with and without heparin. J Reprod Med 37:766-770.

Gynecologic Surgery and Adhesion Prevention, pages 213–220

TISSUE-TYPE PLASMINOGEN ACTIVATOR AND ADHESION PREVENTION

Randall C. Dunn, M.D.
Department of Obstetrics and Gynecology
Baylor College of Medicine
Houston, TX 77030

INTRODUCTION

The pathogenesis of postsurgical adhesion formation has become better understood. Investigators have demonstrated that the production of ischemic tissue after surgical injury by coagulation, ligation or devascularization have all been associated with adhesion formation. (Ellis, 1971; Ellis, 1982) As well, tissue injury by abrasion will also lead to adhesion formation. (Holtz, 1984) After these peritoneal injuries occur, there is a fibrinous exudate released which evolves into a fibrin matrix and becomes early fibrinous adhesions. (Stangel 1984). The ischemic or injured tissue which is left loses its ability to lyse fibrin. (Buckman/Buckman, Buckman/Woods, 1976; Raftery, 1981; Porter, 1969). Additionally, tissue which is rendered ischemic inhibits fibrinolysis by normal adjacent tissue. (Buckman/Buckman, 1976). The majority of early fibrinous adhesions are transient and lysed within 72 hours due to the peritoneal fibrinolytic system (Jackson, 1958). Those fibrinous adhesions which remain become infiltrated by proliferating fibroblasts, followed by vascularization and cellular ingrowth, with resultant permanent adhesion formation. (Holtz, 1984) When fibrinolytic activity is normal the early fibrinous adhesions are lysed and normal peritoneal healing can occur. This has been postulated by animal experiments to be due to depressed plasminogen activator activity. (Buckman/Buckman, 1976; Buckman/Woods, 1976; Diamond/DeCherney, 1987)

Plasmin is the principal agent of the fibrinolytic system. The inactive proenzyme, plasminogen, is converted to plasmin by plasminogen activator. Plasmin then induces fibrinolysis whereever it encounters fibrin and fibrin split products are then formed. (Wiman, 1976; Matsuo, 1981). Plasminogen activators are located in the mesothelium and submesothelial blood vessels. (Porter, 1969) The duration of impaired plasminogen activator activity following serosal injury varies with the type of injury. (Raftery, 1981; Gervin 1973) When plasminogen activator is reduced by 50%, or more, permanent adhesions form. (Gervin, 1973)

PLASMINOGEN ACTIVATORS

Plasminogen activators can be divided into three major categories: Urokinase-type (u-PA), Tissue-type (t-PA), and "Other" types. (Dano, 1985)

u-PA occurs as a one or two chain glycoprotein its active form is a two chain glycoprotein. u-PA's activation of plasminogen can occur both on surface-bound and liquid-phase plasminogen; i.e. on the surface of fibrin and in the plasma, respectively. This activation can cause a high degree of fibrinogenolysis because plasmin is not specific for fibrin degradation alone, but can also bind to its precursor protein, fibrinogen. (Dano, 1985; Matsuo, 1981) u-PA is found in several cell types, but is highest in the genitourinary system. (Dano, 1985)

t-PA also occurs as a one or two chain glycoprotein and is active as a two chain glycoprotein. t-PA is several hundredfold times more effective as an activator of the fibrinolytic system in the presence of fibrin than u-PA. (Ferres, 1987) t-PA's proteolytic activity is confined primarily to the fibrin surface and has little effect on circulating fibrinogen levels. (Ferres, 1987) t-PA is ubiquitous in all tissue homogenates which have been studied. (Ferres, 1987)

"Other" types of plasminogen activators (i.e. streptokinase, coagulation factors XI, XII, kallikrien, etc.) have high degrees of fibrinogenolysis, immunogenicity, and low specific activation potential for fibrinolysis. Streptokinase is a bacterial protein capable of activating plasminogen but its mechanism is completely different. It has no enzymatic activity of its own, but acts by forming an equimolar complex with plasminogen which then has plasminogen activator activity. It too can cause significant fibrinogen degradation. (Ferris, 1987) The coagulation factors XI and XII have a specific plasminogen activator activity less than 10^{-4} of u-PA and do not play a significant physiological role. (Dano, 1985).

Inhibitors of plasminogen activators are ubiquitous and can rapidly neutralize the plasminogen activator's activity. (Dano, 1985) The exact role of plasminogen activator inhibitors is not understood, though a role in fibrinolysis homeostasis is possible. t-PA binds to the fibrin surface and induces proteolytic cleavage of plasminogen to plasmin on the fibrin surface. This sequestration of plasmin after activation by t-PA on the fibrin surface protects it from plasmin's inhibitors allowing for only slow degradation of its fibrinolytic effect. (Matsuo, 1981; Ferris, 1987) In contrast, non-fibrin bound plasmin formed by other activators is rapidly cleared by plasmin inhibitors. (Wiman, 1976).

Since endogenously depressed plasminogen activator activity has been postulated to be the primary factor leading to permanent adhesion formation postsurgically, then the addition of tissue-type plasminogen activator may lead to improved fibrinolysis with subsequent decreased permanent adhesion formation. The experimental evidence from other types of plasminogen activators has been mixed and is reviewed elsewhere. (Dunn, 1991)

EXPERIMENTAL STUDIES

Recently, animal data has been compiled on t-PA's potential as a therapeutic modality to prevent postsurgical adhesions. Recombinant technology has made t-PA commercially available so that studies could be carried out. (Pennica, 1983) Initially, t-PA was formulated into an inert gel and was used in varying dosages to attempt to reduce initial and recurrent postoperative adhesions. The t-PA was shown to be effective in a dose dependent fashion in this rabbit uterine horn abrasion/cautery model. (Doody, 1989) Additional studies in a pelvic uterine horn devascularization model were undertaken to increase the postsurgical ischemic injury to further test t-PA's effectiveness. These were also successful in preventing the formation of postsurgical adhesions. (Dunn, 1990) Approximately three cms of each uterine horn were devascularized by cauterization of their mesenteric vessels and anastomotic branches. Animal's scores were on the basis of the percentage of the total surface of the horns which were involved in adhesion formation. The results are presented in Table 1.

TABLE 1. Results of gel t-PA to prevent postsurgical adhesions. Animals evaluated after 14 days.*

Animals	Score
Control (gel only) (n=14)	21.1
Gel rt-PA (12.5 gms) (n=14)	9.7

*Significance at $p < 0.05$

In a similar rabbit model, adhesions were initially induced by the previously mentioned devascularization injury and after surgical adhesiolysis, gel t-PA was placed topically prior to closure. Results are presented in Table 2. Both groups had similar pre-adhesiolysis adhesion scores.

TABLE 2. t-PA as an adjunct to surgical adhesiolysis. Animals evaluated after 14 days.*

Animals	Score
Control (gel only) (n=13)	51.5
Gel rt-PA (12.5 gms) (n=14)	25.8

*Significance at $p < 0.05$

The effectiveness of topical gel t-PA has been corroborated by other examiners in different animal models. (Mohler, 1987; Menzies, 1989)

To further determine the efficacy of t-PA alone, without any potential mechanical separation effect of the gel delivery vehicle, it was administered postsurgically via an intraperitoneal catheter. Table 3 demonstrates the results when t-PA was administered in liquid form only. Control and treatment groups had liquid infusions every 12 hours for four days. Control groups had diluent only for infusion. Further studies using this model demonstrated an increased effectiveness of t-PA to prevent postsurgical adhesions if the time interval over which the t-PA was infused was increased. This was accomplished despite the fact that the dose at each infusion was less. (Dunn, 1992)

TABLE 3. Effectiveness of liquid t-PA (16 mg total dose) to prevent postsurgical adhesions. Animals evaluated after 10 days.

Animal Groups	Mean Score*	N
Control	35.0	11
Treatment x 4d	3.8	8

*Significance at $p < 0.01$

Similar postive results were also demonstrated with liquid t-PA as an adjunct to surgical adhesiolysis in the prevention of adhesion reformation; see Table 4.

TABLE 4. Mean change in adhesion scores after surgical adhesiolysis using t-PA (16 mg total dose). Animals evaluated after 10 days.

Animal Groups	Mean Score Change*	N
Control	+3	8
Treatment	-28	8

*Significance at $p < 0.02$

Currently, a Phase I trial of liquid t-PA in varying dosages is underway. Safety issues such as the postoperative clinical course, postoperative studies of coagulation parameters and circulating levels of tissue plasminogen activator are being monitored.

CONCLUSIONS

These investigations confirm the importance of the fibrinolytic system as it pertains to postsurgical adhesion formation and reformation. The degree of adhesion formation, and probably adhesion reformation, is related to the degree of initial surgical injury. The absence of peritoneal surface damage remains the hallmark of adhesion-free surgery due to the resulting depression of fibrinolytic activity of the peritoneum due to the depression of plasminogen activator. Maintenance of normal fibrinolytic activity in areas of surgical injury may lead to the resolution of fibrin, and therefore permanent adhesions might not form.

Specific questions regarding the use of these activators still need to be addressed. The variable for time of administration postoperatively remains critical. Current research indicates that from the immediate postoperative time period, up to five days postoperatively, is the critical period that normal fibrinolysis is reduced and intervention helpful. (Buckman/Buckman 1976; Raftery 1981; Diamond/DeCherney 1987; Orita, 1986; Doody 1989; Dunn, 1992). Therefore, a single postoperative dose of tissue plasminogen activator may not be sufficient for adhesion prophylaxis. Future study protocols will need to address this issue so that an adequate trial of tissue plasminogen activator is pursued.

The specific activity of tissue plasminogen activator when administered postoperatively is important due to the possibility of postoperative complications such as altered wound healing or bleeding complications secondary to systemic fibrinolysis and/or fibrinogen consumption. Wound healing complications have as yet to be considered a problem in animal studies. (Doody, 1989; Dunn, 1990) Bleeding complications have also not be seen to be a significant problem. Specifically, when t-PA was utilized in a recent study to prevent adhesion formation and reformation, the circulating levels of t-PA and fibrinogen were assayed and no change in circulating levels was found. (Doody, 1989)

In summary, these data demonstrate that the addition of tissue plasminogen activator postoperatively to prevent adhesion formation/reformation has been successful in animal studies. A Phase I trial of t-PA is underway and future investigations are necessary to determine its effectiveness to handle this important clinical problem.

REFERENCES

Buckman, R.F., Buckman, P.D., Hufnagel, H.W. & Gervin, A.S. (1976). A physiologic basis for the adhesion-free healing of deperitonealized surfaces. J. Surg. Res., 21:67-76.

Buckman, R.F., Woods, M.C., Sargent, L. & Gervin, A.S. (1976). A unifying pathogenetic mechanism in the etiology of intraperitoneal adhesions. J. Surg. Res., 20:1-5.

Dano, K., Andreasen, P.A., Grondahl-Hansen, J., Kristensen, P., Nielsen, L.S. & Skriver, L. (1985). Plasminogen activators, tissue degradation, and cancer. Adv. Can. Res., 44:139-266.

Diamond, M.P. & DeCherney, A.H. (1987). Pathogenesis of adhesion formation/reformation: application to reproductive pelvic surgery. Microsurgery, 8:103-107.

Diamond, M.P., Daniell, J.F., Feste, J., Surrey, M.W., McLaughlin, D.S., Friedman, S., Vaughn, W.K. & Martin, D.C. (1987). Adhesion reformation and de novo adhesion formation after reproductive pelvic surgery. Fertil. Steril., 47(5):864-866.

Doody, K.J., Dunn, R.C. & Buttram, Jr., V.C. (1989). Recombinant tissue plasminogen activator reduces adhesion formation in a rabbit uterine horn model. Fertil. Steril., 51:509-512.

Dunn, R.C. (1991). Adhesions, Adhesiolysis, and Plasminogen Activators. In Hafez, ESE (ed): Assisted Human Reproductive Technology. New York: Hemisphere Publishing Corp., pp. 130-137.

Dunn, R.C. and Mohler, M. (1990). Formation of Adhesions after Surgical Injury and Their Prevention with Tissue-Type Plasminogen Activator in a Rabbit Pelvic Model. Infert., 13:103-111.

Dunn, R.C. and Mohler, M. (1992). Effect of Varying Days of Tissue Plasminogen Activator Therapy on the Prevention of Postsurgical Adhesions in a Rabbit Model. J. Surg. Res. (in review).

Ellis, H. (1962). The aetiology of postoperative adhesions. Br. J. Surg., 50:10-16.

Ellis, H. (1971). The cause and prevention of postoperative intraperitoneal adhesions. Surg. Gynecol. Obstet., 133:497-511.

Ellis, H. (1982). The causes and prevention of intestinal adhesions. Br. J. Surg., 69:241-243.

Ferres, H. (1987). Preclinical pharmacological evaluation of anisoylated plasminogen streptokinase activator complex. Drugs, (Suppl. 3):33-50.

Gervin, A.S., Puchett, G.L. & Silver, D. (1973). Serosal hypofibrinolysis: a cause of postoperative adhesions. Am. J. Surg., 125:80-88.

Holtz, G. (1984). Prevention and management of peritoneal adhesions. Fertil. Steril., 41:497-507.

Jackson, B.B. (1958). Observations on intraperitoneal adhesions: an experimental study. Surg., 44:507-514.

James, D.C.O., Ellis, H. & Hugh, T.B. (1965). The effect of streptokinase on experimental intraperitoneal adhesions formation. J. Path. Bact., 90:279-287.

Jewett, T.C., Ambrus, J. & Ambrus, C. (1965). Effects of fibrinolytic enzymes on experimentally induced peritoneal adhesions. Surg., 27:280-284.

Matsuo, O., Rijken, D.C. & Collen, D. (1981). Comparison of the relative fibrinogenolytic, fibrinolytic and thrombolytic properties of tissue plasminogen activator and urokinase in vitro. Thrombos. Haemostas., 45:225-229.

Meier, H., Dietl, K.H. & Willital, G.H. (1985). Initial clinical results of the prevention in intraoperative adhesions in children. Langenbecks Arch. Chir., 366:191-193.

Milligan, D.W. & Raftery, A.T. (1974). Observations on the pathogenesis of peritoneal adhesions: a light and electron microscopical study. Br. J. Surg., 61:274-280.

Mohler, M., Hollenbach, S., Nguyen, T., Reger, V., Hotchkiss, A. (1987). Effect of Recombinant Tissue-Type Plasminogen Activator (rt-PA) on the Prevention of Intraabdominal Adhesion Formation. Thrombos. Haemostas 58(1):270.

Mund-Hoym, S., Roberg, A. & Schander, K. (1984). Prevention of postoperative adhesions-an animal study. Geburtsh u Frauenheilk., 44:463-467.

Orita, H., Campeau, J.D., Gale, J.A., Nakamura, R.M. & diZerega, G.S. (1986). Differential secretion of plasminogen activator activity by postsurgical activated macrophages. J. Surg. Res., 41:569-573.

Pennica, D., Holmes, W.E., Kohr, W.J., Harkins, R.N., Vehar, G.A., Ward, C.A., Bennett, W.F., Yelverton, E., Seeburg, P.H., Heyneker, H.L., Goeddel, D.V. & Collen, D. (1983). Cloning and expression of human tissue-type plasminogen activator cDNA in E. Coli. Nature, 301:214-221.

Porter, J.M., McGregor, F.H., Mullin, D.C. & Silver, D. (1969). Fibrinolytic activity of mesothelial surfaces. Surg. Forum, 20:80-82.

Raftery, A.T. (1981). Effect of peritoneal trauma on peritoneal fibrinolytic activity and intraperitoneal adhesion formation. An experimental study in the rat. Eur. Surg. Res., 13:397-401.

Rivkind, A.I., Lieberman, N. & Durst, A.L. (1985). Urokinase does not prevent abdominal adhesion formation in rats. Eur. Surg. Res., 17:254-258.

Shimanuki, T., Nakamura, R.M. & diZerega, G.S. (1986). A kinetic analysis of peritoneal fluid cytology and arachidonic acid metabolism after abrasion and reabrasion of rabbit peritoneum. J. Surg. Res., 41:245-251.

Stangel, J.J., Nisbet II, J.D., & Settles, H. (1984). Formation and prevention of postoperative abdominal adhesions. J. Reprod. Med., 29:143-156.

Thomas, J.W., Greene, J.W. & Rhoads, J.E. (1950). An experimental study of factors affecting the development and persistence of intraperitoneal fibrous adhesions. Surg. Forum, 1:125-127.

Wiman, B. & Collen, D. (1978). Molecular mechanism of physiological fibrinolysis. Nature, 272:549-550.

Wright, L.T., Smith, D.H., Rothman, M., Quash, E.T. & Metzger, W.I. (1950). Prevention of postoperative adhesions in rabbits with streptococcal metabolites. Proc. Soc. Exp. Biol. Med., 75:602-604.

Gynecologic Surgery and Adhesion Prevention, pages 221–233

USE OF INTERCEED (TC7) ABSORBABLE ADHESION BARRIER TO REDUCE POSTOPERATIVE ADHESION FORMATION IN INFERTILITY AND ENDOMETRIOSIS SURGERY

Kaoru Sekiba, M.D.
OB/GYN Adhesion Prevention Committee, Japan
Department of Obstetrics and Gynecology
Okayama University Medical School
2-5-1 Shikata, Okayama 700, Japan

Peritoneal adhesions are one of the major causes of chronic or recurrent pelvic pain [Rapkin(1986), Malinak(1980)], and recognized as a major cause of infertility [Drake(1980)]. Endometriosis is a common cause of pelvic adhesions. Both medical and surgical therapies are utilized to treat endometriosis. A major limitation of surgical treatment is postoperative adhesion formation. Lysis of these adhesions is usually followed by recurrence of the adhesions [Jansen(1988), Luciano(1987, 1989), Trimbos-Kemper(1986), Tulandi(1986)]. Both microsurgical and Laparoscopic approaches have been used to reduce formation of postoperative adhesions. Recently, an oxidized regenerated cellulose barrier, INTERCEED(TC7), was reported to reduce formation of pelvic adhesions in patients undergoing infertility surgery [INTERCEED(TC7) Adhesion Barrier Study Group(1989)]. Although a benefit was shown in that study, no data were available which addressed the patients with extensive endometriosis. Here we report the utility of INTERCEED(TC7) to prevent the reformation of postoperative adhesions after infertility surgery including those patients with severe endometriosis.

Principal investigators and study sites were: Kaoru Sekiba, M.D. and Nobutaka Yoshida, M.D., Department of Obstetrics and Gynecology, Okayama University Medical School, Okayama, Okayama; Takao Fukaya, M.D., Department of Obstetrics and Gynecology, Tohoku University School of Medicine, Sendai, Miyagi; Tsutomu Ono, M.D., Department of Obstetrics and Gynecology, Yamagata University School of Medicine, Yamagata, Yamagata; Hideki Mizunuma, M.D.,

Department of Obstetrics and Gynecology School of Medicine, Gunma University, Maebashi, Gunma; Hisao Osada, M.D., Department of Obstetrics and Gynecology, Nihon University School of Medicine, Itabashi, Tokyo; Naoki Mitsuhashi, M.D., Department of Obstetrics and Gynecology, Faculty of Medicine, University of Tokyo, Bunkyo, Tokyo; Kazuo Sugimura, M.D., Department of Obstetrics and Gynecology, School of Medicine, Keio University, Shinjuku, Tokyo; Hideo Awaji, M.D., Department of Obstetrics and Gynecology, School of Medicine, Tokai University, Isehara, Kanagawa; Tomio Sawada, M.D., Department of Obstetrics and Gynecology, Fujita-Gakuen Health University, Toyoake, Aichi; Yoichi Noda, M.D., Department of Gynecology and Obstetrics, Faculty of Medicine, Kyoto University, Kyoto, Kyoto; Kazunori Miyazaki, M.D., Department of Obstetrics and Gynecology, Osaka Medical College, Takatsuki, Osaka; and Fumitaka Saji, M.D., Department of Obstetrics and Gynecology, Osaka University Medical School, Osaka, Osaka.

MATERIALS AND METHODS

Sixty-three infertility patients in 12 investigational centers participated in this randomized study. The study protocol was approved by ethical review in each study center. All were over 18 years of age, had both tubes and ovaries, and bilateral pelvic sidewall adhesions. Patients with hemorrhagic or coagulation disorders, pelvic infection or pregnancy were excluded. At laparotomy they received no other treatment for adhesion prevention including 32% Dextran 70, peritoneal grafts or fibrin glue. Postoperative hydrotubation was not performed.

After completion of all operative procedures including lysis of pelvic sidewall adhesions, the area of the denuded peritoneal surface was measured over the pelvic sidewall using a sterile ruler. A sealed envelope was opened which identified, on a randomized basis, the pelvic sidewall to be covered with INTERCEED(TC7). INTERCEED(TC7) was applied in an amount sufficient to completely cover all deperitonealized surfaces on the indicated pelvic sidewall and leave a border between the perimeter of injury and the edge of INTERCEED(TC7). INTERCEED(TC7) was supplied as a sterile unit of 7.6 x 10.2 cm by Johnson & Johnson Medical K.K., Tokyo, Japan. INTERCEED(TC7) was placed dry on the deperitonealized surface, and sufficient irrigation solution (2-5mL) was applied to moisten the barrier. As a result, INTERCEED(TC7) adhered to the peritoneal sidewall without suturing. The locations of adhesions and pelvic sidewall areas involved with adhesions were recorded on standardized forms. Photographs were taken and drawing were made to document operative findings. Severity of endometriosis was recorded according to the revised American Fertility Society classification [The American Fertility Society (1985)].

The incidence of adhesion reformation along the pelvic sidewalls was assessed at laparoscopy performed between 10 days and 14 weeks after laparotomy. At the time of laparoscopy, the investigator performing the laparoscopy was unaware of the assignment of sidewall treatment. Data were recorded in a similar manner and compared to the findings at laparotomy. When adhesions were present along the pelvic sidewall atudy site, their area was measured at laparoscopy using a calibrated prove. Reduction of adhesions was expressed as: (1) area differential = deperitonealized area at laparotomy - re-adhesion area at laparoscopy, and (2) percent improvement = (area differential / deperitonealized area at laparotomy) x 100. The effectiveness of these data was analyzed by paired t-test, t-test, chi-square and McNemar's test. Since patients served as their own controls, the paired t-test and McNemar's test were useful to assess treatment effect. $P<0.05$ indicated statistical significance.

RESULTS

Patients ages ranged between 18 and 41 years, with a mean of 30.8 years. Forty-six patients (73%) were nulligravida. The causes of pelvic adhesions included prior infections (nine cases), prior surgery (15 cases), endometriosis (28 cases) and unknown causes (19 cases). Endometriosis was found in 32 patients. The severity of endometriosis was: class I two cases; class II two cases; class III eight cases; and class IV 20 cases.

Application of INTERCEED(TC7) was randomized to the right sidewall in 34 (54%) of the patients and to the left sidewall in 29 (46%). The INTERCEED(TC7)-treated sidewalls contained significantly fewer adhesions than the control sidewalls ($P<0.0001$; Figure 1). In 25 patients, the control sidewalls contained adhesions while the INTERCEED(TC7)-treated sidewalls did not have adhesions. In contrast, in three patients adhesions were present on the INTERCEED(TC7) -treated sidewall while no adhesions were present on the control sidewall. This effect of INTERCEED(TC7) in preventing adhesion reformation was shown by matched-pair analysis to be significantly different ($P<0.0001$). When adhesions formed, the INTERCEED(TC7)-treated sidewalls had significantly less area involved with adhesions compared with the control side ($P<0.01$; Figure 2).

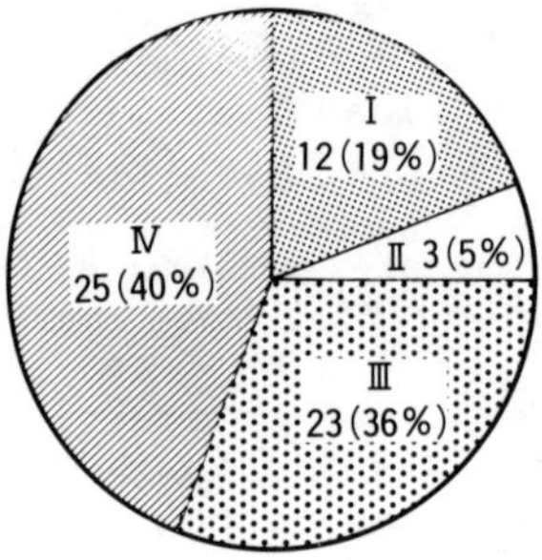

	I	II	III	IV
INTERCEED (TC7)	−	+	+	−
Control	−	−	+	+

+ : Adhesion Present
− : Adhesion Absent

Figure 1

Matched-Pair comparison of the incidence (absence/presence) of sidewall adhesions at laparoscopy (n=63). In 24% of the cases (I+II), the control sidewalls did not contain adhesions. In contrast, in 59% of the cases (I+IV), INTERCEED (TC7)-treated sidewalls had no adhesions (P<0.0001, χ^2 Test). In a matched-sidewall comparison, INTERCEED (TC7) was eight times more effective than control (25 versus 3, P<0.0001, McNemar Test).

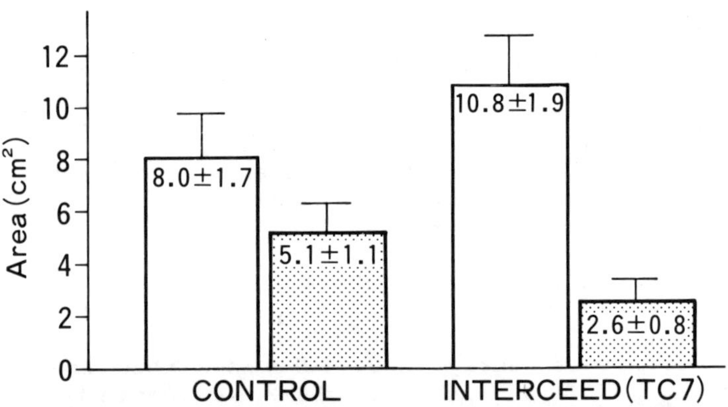

Figure 2

Deperitonealized areas of both pelvic sidewalls in each patient at laparotomy (n=63, mean±SEM, opened bars) are shown. At follow up laparoscopy, the area involved with adhesions (dotted bars) was significantly less for pelvic sidewalls covered by INTERCEED (TC7) at laparotomy (P<0.01, paired t-test).

The 205 individual deperitonealized areas for all sidewalls were divided into two groups (sutured and non-sutured group). In the control sidewalls, the sutured group (33 of 61 or 54%) had significantly fewer areas involved with adhesions than the non-sutured group (31 of 42 or 74%) at laparoscopy ($P<0.05$; Figure 3). In the sutured group, the INTERCEED(TC7)-treated sidewalls (14 of 43 or 33%) had significantly fewer areas involved with adhesions than the control sidewalls at laparoscopy ($P<0.05$; Figure 3). In the non-sutured group, the INTERCEED(TC7)-treated sidewalls (16 of 59 or 27%) had significantly fewer areas involved with adhesions than the control sidewalls at laparoscopy ($P<0.00001$; Figure 3). The percent improvment of the control sidewalls increased by the suturing of peritoneum. In conetrast the percent improvement of the INTERCEED(TC7)-treated sidewalls was fewer and similar in these two groups(Figure 4).

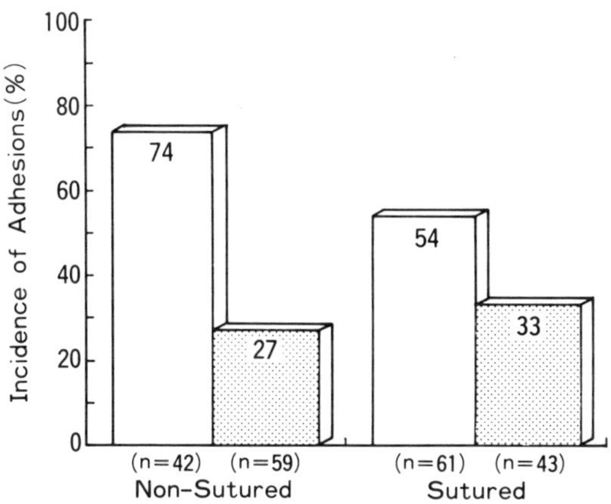

Figure 3

Each of the deperitonealized areas for all sidewalls were divided into two groups (non-sutured and sutured group). On the control sidewalls (opened bars), the sutured group was less involved with adhesions than the non-sutured groups ($P<0.05$, χ^2 Test). But even the sutured group contained adhesions in over 50% of the sites. However, the INTERCEED(TC7)-treated sidewalls (dotted bars) had significantly fewer areas involved with adhesions than the control sidewalls in non-sutured ($P<0.00001$, χ^2 Test) and sutured ($P<0.05$, χ^2 Test) groups.

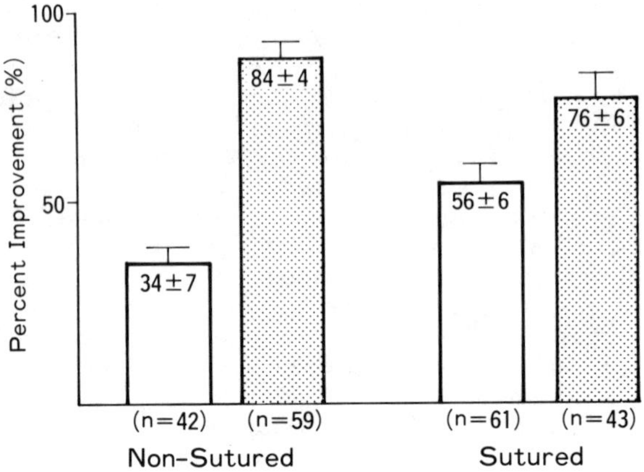

Figure 4

The percent improvement of adhesions in non-sutured and sutured groups. Improvement was significantly better for the INTERCEED(TC7)-treated sidewalls (dotted bars) compared to control sidewalls (opened bars) in non-sutured ($P<0.001$, student t-test) and sutured($P<0.05$, student t-test) groups(mean±SEM).

The 205 individual deperitonealized areas for all sidewalls were divided into three groups (less than $100mm^2$, n=72; $100mm^2$-$1000mm^2$, n=95; more than $1000mm^2$, n=38). In the smallest areas(group I), the INTERCEED(TC7)-treated sidewalls (7 of 35 or 20%) had significantly less areas involved with adhesions than the control sidewalls (17 of 37 or 46%) at laparoscopy($P<0.05$; Figure 5). In the intermediate group (II), the INTERCEED(TC7)-treated sidewalls (12 of 44 or 27%) had significantly fewer areas involved with adhesions than the control sidewalls (32 of 51 or 63%) at laparoscopy ($P<0.01$). In the group with the largest areas (III), the INTERCEED(TC7)-treated sidewalls (11 of 23 or 48%) had significantly fewer areas involved with adhesions than the control sidewalls (15 of 15) at laparoscopy ($P<0.001$). The percent improvement of the control sidewalls decreased as the initial extent of adhesions increased (Figure 6). In contrast, the percent improvement of the INTERCEED(TC7)-treated sidewalls was similar in all groups.

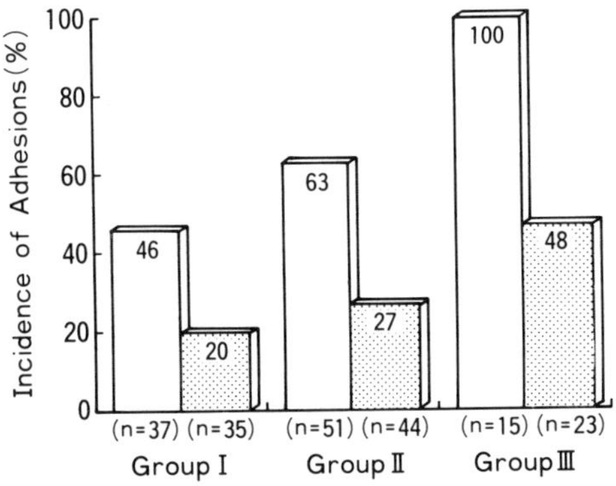

Figure 5

Each of the deperitonealized areas (DAs) for all sidewalls were divided into three groups (group I: DA<100mm^2, n=72; group II: 100mm^2≦DA<1000mm^2, n=95; group III: 1000mm^2≦DA, n=38). On the control sidewalls (opened bars), the incidence of adhesions at laparoscopy increased as size of the deperitonealized areas increased (P<0.005, χ^2 Test). The INTERCEED(TC7)-treated sidewalls (dotted bars) had significantly fewer areas involved with adhesions than the control sidewalls on the each group (group I: P<0.05; group II:P<0.001; group III: P<0.001, χ^2 Test).

Twenty eight patients had severe endometriosis (class III and IV). Significantly fewer INTERCEED(TC7)-treated sidewalls contained adhesions (with adhesions 14 of 28 cases or 50%) than on the control side (with adhesions 23 of 28 cases or 82%; P<0.05). In nine women, adhesions were present on the control side while no adhesions were present on the INTERCEED(TC7)-treated sidewall. In no patient were adhesions present on the INTERCEED(TC7)-treated sidewalls when adhesions were not present on the control sidewalls. These results show that in patients with severe endometriosis, significantly more pelvic sidewalls treated with INTERCEED(TC7) did not have adhesions compared to control sidewalls (P<0.01; Figure 7). In cases of severe endometriosis, the percent improvement of deperitonealized

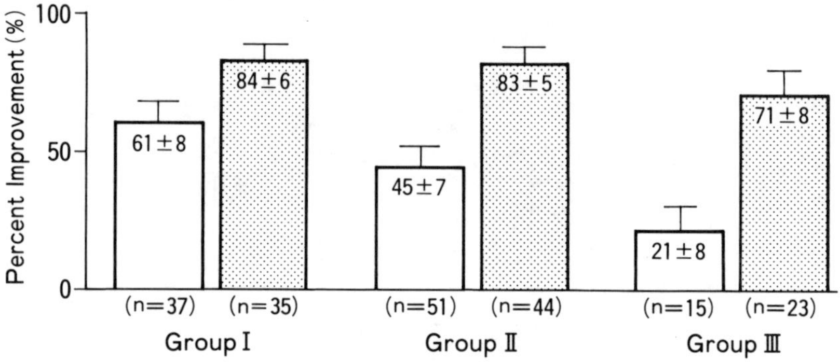

Figure 6

The percent improvement of adhesions for three deperitonealized areas groups (reference: Figure 5). The percent improvement of the deperitonealized areas (DAs) of INTERCEED(TC7)-treated sidewalls were similar (mean±SEM, dotted bars). In contrast, the percent improvement of the control sidewalls decreased as the initial extent of adhesions increased (opened bars)(group I: $P<0.05$; group II: $P<0.001$; group III: $P<0.001$, student t-test).

area of INTERCEED(TC7)-treated sidewalls was also significantly greater than that of control sidewalls ($P<0.001$; Figure 8).

Thirty one patients without endometriosis were studied. On the INTERCEED(TC7)-treated side significantly less adhesions were observed (with adhesions 12 of 31 cases or 39%) than on the control side (with adhesions 22 of 31 cases or 71%; $P<0.05$). In 13 patients, adhesions were present on the control side while no adhesions were present on the INTERCEED(TC7)-treated sidewalls. In contrast, in three patients adhesions were present on the INTERCEED(TC7)-treated sidewalls while no adhesions were present on the control sidewalls. Using matched-pair analysis significantly more INTERCEED(TC7)-treated sidewalls did not have adhesions compared to the control sidewalls ($P<0.05$; Figure 7). When adhesions formed, the percent improvement of deperitonealized area of INTERCEED(TC7)-treated sidewalls was significantly greater than that of control sidewalls ($P<0.001$; Figure 8).

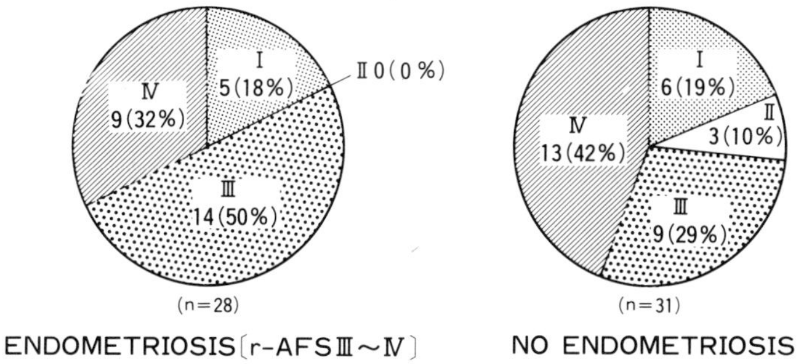

	I	II	III	IV
INTERCEED(TC7)	−	+	+	−
Control	−	−	+	+

+ : Adhesion Present
− : Adhesion Absent

Figure 7

Matched-Pair comparioson of the incidence (absence/presence) of sidewall adhesions at laparoscopy with and without severe endometriosis (American Fertility Society revised classification class III and IV). Using Matched-Pair analysis significantly more INTERCEED(TC7)-treated sidewalls did not have adhesions compared to the control sidewalls in patients with [50%(I+IV) vs. 18%(I+II),P<0.05, χ^2 Test] and without [61%(I+IV) vs. 29%(I+II), P<0.05, χ^2 Test] endometriosis.

DISCUSSION

Previously a clinical evaluation of INTERCEED(TC7) as a surgical adjuvant to reduce the formation of pelvic adhesions was reported by the Adhesion Barrier Study Group (1989). In that report INTERCEED(TC7) was shown to be four times more effective in preventing adhesion reformation than surgery alone in a matched comparison of pelvic sidewalls within the same patient. Here, we confirm and extend the previous findings. In the present study, INTERCEED(TC7) was eight times more effective than surgery alone in preventing adhesion formation. Why did the present study demonstrate a greater benefit from INTERCEED(TC7) than the previous report? In the North American study, INTERCEED(TC7) efficacy

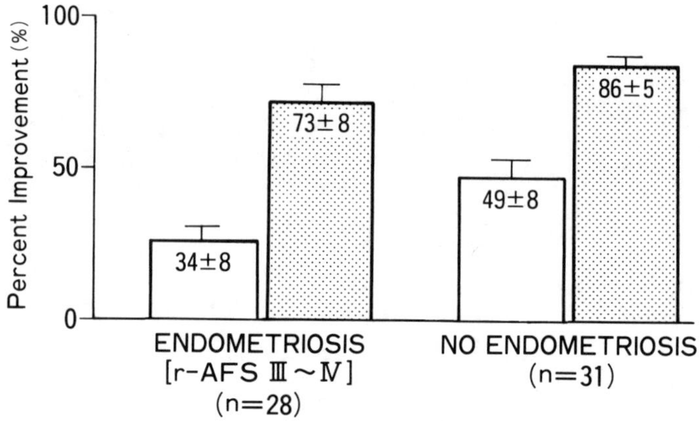

Figure 8

Percent improvement of adhesions in pelvic sidewalls with and without severe endometriosis (American Fertility Society revised classification class III and IV). Improvement was siginificantly better for sidewalls treated with INTERCEED(TC7) (dotted bars) compared to surgery alone (opened bars) in patients with ($P<0.001$, paired t-test) and without ($P<0.001$, paired t-test) endometriosis (mean±SEM)

depended on good hemostasis at the primary site of surgery, as well as removal of peritoneal instillates prior to barrier application. In the present study, strict attention was paid to these technical details. In addition, coverage of the deperitonealized site with INTERCEED(TC7) was sufficient to extend well beyond the perimeter of the surgical injury. In this way, potential areas of peri-surgical inflammation were covered thereby allowing for a clear discrimination of treatment effect.

In the current study, 28 patients had severe endometriosis on the basis of the American Fertility Society classification. This is the first report using INTERCEED(TC7) barrier to prevent adhesions after surgical treatment of severe endometriosis. Resection of severe endometriosis usually leads to adhesion formation as shown in this study by an 82% incidence of control sidewalls with adhesions. However, use of INTERCEED(TC7) barrier resulted in prevention of adhesion in 50% of the sidewalls.

In this study, the deperitonealized areas on all sidewalls were divided into three groups from small to large depending on the size of the initial areas. On the control sidewalls, the percent improvement decreased as size of the deperitonealized areas increased. In contrast, the percent improvement of INTERCEED(TC7)-treated areas were uniform regardless of the initial extent of injury. Accordingly, these results show that INTERCEED(TC7) prevented adhesion reformation regardless of the initial size of the deperitonealied area.

Tulandi [Tulandi (1988)] reported that suturing of peritoneum actually increased the incidence of adhesions. But we could not confirm these results. On the control sidewalls, the sutured group was less involved with adhesions than the non-sutured group. But even the sutured group contained adhesions in over 50% of the sites. However, since the INTERCEED(TC7)-treated sidewalls were involved with fewer areas of adhesion than the control sidewalls, these results show that suturing is not necessary at the time of INTERCEED(TC7) application.

Animal studies show that mechanical barriers can prevent adhesion formation by limiting tissue apposition during the initial phases of peritoneal repair [Soules (1982)]. In the initial clinical study, performed in the United States, 32% Dextran 70 was found to have limited benefit in reducing formation of postsurgical pelvic adhesions [Adhesion Study Group (1983)]. This was not confirmed in a follw up study performed in Sweden using the same protocol [Larsson (1985)] nor in a subsequent study of infertility patients performed in Australia [Jansen(1985)]. Chondroitin sulfate [Oelsner (1987)] and carboxymethyl cellulose [Diamond (1988); Elkins,(1984a, 1984b, 1985); Fredericks (1986)], also barrier solutions, show potential for postsurgical adhesion prevention in animal models. In none of the above reports are studies of postsurgical adhesion prevention available in cases of severe endometriosis. The polytetrafluoroethylen barrier (Gore-Tex) [Boyers (1988)] was shown to reduce the formation of post surgical pelvic adhesions in a rabbit uterine horn model. This result was not confirmed in a similar animal study [Goldberg(1987)]. Gore-Tex must be sutured in place, is permanent, and can not expand when used to cover the uterus.

In conclusion, INTERCEED(TC7) readily adheres to deperitonealized areas then rapidly forms a soft gelatinous mass which protects tissues during re-epithelialization. INTERCEED(TC7) absorbable adhesion barrier can prevent reformation of postsurgical adhesions after infertility surgery including patients with severe endometriosis and those with large areas of deperitonealization.

REFERENCES

Adhesion study Group (1983). Reduction of postoperative pelvic adhesions with intraperitoneal 32% dextran 70: a prospective, randomized clinical trial. Fertil Steril 40:612-9

Boyers SP, Diamond MP, DaCherenay AH (1988). Reduction of postoperative pelvic adhesions in the rebbit with Gore-Tex surgical membrane. Fertil Steril 49: 1066-70

Diamond MP, DaCherney AH, Linsky CB, Cunningham T, Constantine B (1988). Adhesion Re-formation in the rabbit uterine horn model: 1.Reduction with carboxymethyl cellulose. Int J Infertil 33: 372-5

Drake TS, Grunert GM, (1980). The unsuspected pelvic factor in the infertility investigation. Fertil Steril 34:27-31

Elkins TE, Bury RJ, Ritter JL, et al (1984a). Adhesion prevention by solution of sodium carboxymethyl cellulose in the rat, I. Fertil Steril 41: 926-8

Elkins TE, Ling FW, Ahokas RA, Abdella TN, Homsey CA, Malinak LR (1984b). Adhesion prevention by solution of sodium carboxymethylcellulose in the rat, II. Fertil Steril 41:929-32

Elkins TE, Trenthem L, McNeely SG-Jr, FW, prewitt J, Homsey CA, Malinak LR (1985). Potential for in vitro growth of common bacteria in solutions of 32% dextran 70 and 1.0% odium carboxymethylcellulose. Fertil Steril 43: 477-8

Fredericks CM, Kotry I, Holz G et al (1986). Adhesion prevention in the rabbit with sodium carboxymethyl cellulose solutions. Am J Obstet Gynecol 155: 667-70

Goldberg JM, Toledo AA, Mitchel DE (1987). An evalution of the Gore-Tex surgical mambrane for the prevention of Postoperative oeritoneal adhesions. Obetet Gynecol 70:846-8

INTERCEED(TC7) Adhesion Barrier Study Group (1989). Prevention of postsurgical adhesions by INTERCEED(TC7), an absorbable adhesion barrier : prospective, randomized multicenter clinical study. Fertil Steril 51: 933-938

Jansen RPS (1985). Failure of intraperitoneal adjuncts to improve the outcome of pelvic operations in young women. Am J Obstet Gynecol 153: 363-71

Jansen RPS (1988). Early laparoscopy after pelvic operations to prevent adhesions: safety and efficacy. Fertil Steril 49: 26-31

Larsson B, Lalos O, Marsk L et al (1985). Effect of intraperitoneal instillation of 32% dextran 70 on postoperative adhesion formation after tubal surgery. Acta Obstet Gynecol Scand 64: 437-41

Luciano AA, Whitman G, Maier DB, Randolph J, Maenze R (1987). A Comparison of thermal injury healing patterns, and postoperative adhesion formation following CO_2 laser and electromicrosurgery. Fertil Steril 48 : 1025-9

Luciano AA, Maier DB, Koch EI, Nulsen JC (1989). A comparative study of postoperative adhesions following laser surgery by laparoscopy versus laparotomy in the rabbit model. Obstet Gynecol 74: 220-4

Malinak LR, Operative managemant of pelvic pain (1980). Clin Obstet Gynecol 23: 191-200

Malinak LR (1990). INTERCEED(TC7) as an adjuvant for adhesion reduction: clinical studies. In: diZerega GS, Malinak LR, Diamond MP, and Linsky CB eds. Treatment of Post surgical Adhesions (Progress in clinical and biological research Vol. 358) New York: Wiley-Liss 193-206

Oelsner G, Graebe RA, Pan S-B, et al (1987). Chondroitin Sulphate. A new intraperitoneal treatme for postoperative adhesion prevention in the rabbit. J Reprod Med32:812-4

Rapkin A (1986). Adhesion and Pelvic pain, UCLA. Obstet Gynecol68:13-5

Soules MR, Dennis L, Bosarge A, Moore DE(1982). The Prevention of postoperative pelvic adhesions: An animal study comparing barrier methods with dextran 70. Am J obstet Gynecol 143 : 829-34

The American Fertility Society (1985). Revised American Fertility Society classification of endometriosis 1985 FertilSteril43:351-5

Trimbos-Kemper TCM, Trimbos JB, Van Hall EV (1985). Adhesion formation after tubal surgery: results of the eighth-day laparoscopy in 188 patients. Fertil Steril 43: 395-400

Tulandi T (1986). Salpingo-Ovariolysis: a comparison between laser surgery and electrosurgery. Fertil Steril 45: 489-91

Tulandi T, Hum HS, Gelfand, MM (1988). Closure of laparotomy incisions with or without peritoneal suturing and second-look laparoscopy. Am J Obstet Gynecol 158: 536-7

Gynecologic Surgery and Adhesion Prevention, pages 235–251

NEW MODALITIES UNDER DEVELOPMENT FOR ADHESION PREVENTION: IMMUNOMODULATORY AGENTS AND POLOXAMER BARRIER MATERIALS

Alex Steinleitner, M.D.
Hovey Lambert, Ph.D.
Simon Henderson, M.D., D.Phil.
San Francisco Center for Reproductive Medicine
and the Department of Obstetrics and Gynecology
California Pacific Medical Center
San Francisco, CA 94118

INTRODUCTION

Adhesion reformation remains the most important problem facing reproductive surgeons in the 1990's. Despite a decade's attention to atraumatic microsurgical technique, the development of a variety of adhesion prevention adjuvants, and the introduction of laser surgical technology, adhesion reformation following lysis of thick established adhesive bands is the rule and not the exception.

Why does the body resist the surgeon's best efforts at surgical reconstruction? From a teleologic standpoint, homeostasis is the organism's primary concern. The body is always prepared for a worst case scenario. To "live to fight another day" after major trauma, homeostatic systems are in place that aggressively fight bacterial infection, promptly staunch bleeding from open vessels and abraded tissues, phagocytize damaged tissues, and rapidly synthesize resilient tissue to repair the injured organ.

Although this may be a life-saving sequence of events following a knife or gunshot wound, this "all out" response diametrically opposes the goals of the infertility surgeon. In the course of excising adhesions with surgically precise incisions, the surgeon is attempting to influence healing in the direction of reperitonealization with restoration of normal anatomic relationships. Unfortunately, the patient's homeostatic mechanisms are not aware of the surgeon's intentions. Relatively mild tissue injury may result in the production of inflammatory mediators that may activate components of the adhesion formation cascade.

In this review we will touch briefly on the pathophysiology of peritoneal wound repair and summarize studies evaluating immunomodulatory agents designed to favorably influence aspects of postsurgical healing. Additionally, we will describe preclinical studies developing a unique new barrier material for infertility surgery.

PHYSIOLOGY OF PERITONEAL REPAIR

Peritoneal repair is recognized to be an integrated, dynamic process. Current evidence suggests that the peritoneal macrophage has an important role in the regulation of the events of each phase of the mesothelial repair process. The degree to which inflammatory stimuli activate postsurgical peritoneal macrophages is thought to be a critical determinate of the ultimate outcome of mesothelial healing (Riches, 1988). An understanding of the various means through which the peritoneal macrophage directs the cellular elements participating in repair is essential to the design of adhesion prevention regimens. These events may be summarized as follows:

Acute postinjury phase - Tissue injury associated with surgical trauma promotes the production and release of factors (leukotriene B_4, complement factor C5a, formyl methionyl peptides, collagen and fibrinonectin fragments) which attract peritoneal macrophages and peripheral monocytes to the wound surface. Exposure to interferons primes macrophages for subsequent activation by factors such as lipopolysaccharide (Murray, et al, 1985).

The activated macrophage is involved both directly and indirectly in the acute postinjury phase of healing. Activated macrophages participate in tissue debridement and bacteriostasis through the production of toxic oxygen radicals and proteolytic enzymes (plasminogen activator, collagenase, elastase) and the phagocytosis of connective tissue matrix (Hensen and Johnston, 1987). Secretion of tumor necrosis factor (TNF) by activated macrophages increases microvascular permeability, augmenting histamine-induced transudation of fibrin rich plasma as substrate for clot formation.

The activated postsurgical macrophage directs the

activities of other cellular elements through the production of soluble factors. Fibroblast collagenase synthesis, an integral event of early tissue remodeling, is markedly stimulated by a macrophage derived factor, tentatively identified as interleukin-1 (IL-1)(Postlethwaite et al, 1983). Granuloycte-mediated tissue phagocytosis and bacteriostasis is directed by macrophage-derived factors, principally TNF and IL-1.

The activation of granulocytes (principally polymorphonuclear leukocytes [PMNs]) is a critical determinate of postsurgical tissue injury. Granulocytes serve as the effector cell for macrophage-directed bacteriostasis and tissue phagocytosis during the acute postinjury phase of healing. PMNs constitute the predominate inflammatory cell type during the initial 24 hours following peritoneal injury (Raftery, 1973). At this juncture granulocytes may play a beneficial role by combating bacterial infection. However, high local concentrations of granulocyte chemotatic and activating factors may evoke enhanced PMN demargination and migration to the site of injury, resulting in granulocyte hyperactivation and extensive phagocytic injury to viable peritoneal surfaces.

Cytokine-mediated activation of PMNs stimulates increased endothelial cell adhesiveness (Bevilacqua et al, 1985) and aggregation (Craddock et al, 1977). Consequently granulocytes undergo marked alterations in their hemorheologic properties (Schmid-Schönbein et al, 1980). Activated granulocytes entering terminal capillary beds are too large and adhesive to transit the system, and thus cause capillary plugging and microvascular ischemia (Schmid-Schönbein, 1987). Primed granulocytes are also known to effect direct microvascular injury to endothelial cells (Harlan, 1987). Subsequent reperfusion injury (McCord, 1987) may result in a degree of injury out of proportion to the macrosurgically evident trauma.

Platelet activation, platelet-endothelial cell interaction, and thrombosis are commonly overlooked, but essential contributors to posttraumatic peritoneal injury. Platelet activation following tissue disruption results in the release of chemotatic and inflammatory mediators (platelet derived growth factor [PDGF], thromboxane A_2, platelet factor 4 [PF4], transforming growth factor ß). Potential mechanisms for platelet-derived mediator initiated peritoneal injury include: 1) increased nonspecific phagocytic damage, 2) enhanced neutrophil adhesiveness for endothelial cells, resulting in microvascular plugging and subsequent reperfusion injury, and 3) unchecked local thrombosis resulting in microvascular shunting of perfusion away from the site of injury.

Prostacyclin (PGI), a product of the cyclooxygenase pathway of prostaglandin synthesis, is an essential regulator of vascular tone, platelet function, and thrombosis following vascular injury. Platelet activation in response to most known stimulants is dramatically inhibited by PGI in vivo. Vascular elaboration of PGI may reduce nonspecific phagocytic tissue injury by inhibiting the production of inflammatory cell chemotatic and activating factors and by ameliorating inflammatory cell activation. PGI has been suggested to have "cytoprotective" properties in a variety of organ injury states (Bursch and Schulte-Hermann, 1987), postulated to be the result of cell membrane protection from free radical production (Thiemermann et al, 1984).

Fibrinolysis - Lysis of fibrinous matrices enveloping adjacent organs is a critical step in the reestablishment of normal peritoneal continuity. Buckman, et al (1976) has shown that the principal determinate of the efficiency of fibrinolysis is the extent to which tissue plasminogen activator (tPA) production by peritoneal surfaces is inhibited by phagocytic injury suffered during the acute postinjury phase of healing. Incomplete fibrinolysis provides a framework of clot matrices for cellularization by fibroblasts and neovascular elements, leading to the formation of dense fibrotic adhesions encasing abdominal viscera. Fibrinolysis is influenced by peritoneal macrophages both indirectly via the regulation of the extent of granulocyte-mediated phagocytic tissue injury and directly through the production of tPA by macrophages which have penetrated clot matrices.

Reperitonealization - The final stage of repair, reperitonealization, is initiated four to seven days after injury by the proliferation of subperitoneal mesenchymal cells arising from the base of the wound. This process is influenced by macrophages via the secretion of ground matrix components, angiogenesis factors, monokines, and growth factors (Fukasawa, et al, 1989, Hunt, et al, 1984, Martin, et al, 1981). Under optimal circumstances this process yields mesothelial surfaces indistinguishable from native peritoneum. Severe tissue injury and ischemia is thought to alter this progression of events. Secretion of macrophage-derived mediators may be augmented to promote the ingrowth of neovascular elements and myofibroblasts into fibrinous matrices in an attempt to restore perfusion to damaged structures (Knighton, et al, 1981, 1983). IL-1 (Schmidt, et al, 1984), macrophage-derived growth factor (Liebvoich and Ross, 1976), angiogenesis factor (Polverni, et al, 1977) have been implicated in this process. The precise contribution of these factors, their sequence of production, and the effect of macrophage activation on mediator production remain to be elucidated.

Platelet activation leads to the release growth factors thought to affect the kinetics of reperitonealization. PDGF, PF4, connective tissue activating peptide III, ß-thromboglobulin, and epidermal growth factor are potent fibroblast chemotactins and stimulants of fibroblast proliferation and collagen deposition. Excessive growth factor release following platelet activation may produce an aberrant stimulus for fibroblast proliferation into fibrin matrices. This process may lead to cellularization of fibrinous adhesions binding adjacent intraperitoneal structures and the formation of dense cellular intraperitoneal adhesions.

IMMUNOMODULATORY AGENTS IN ADHESION PREVENTION

Researchers studying problems in mesothelial healing have recognized that the course of peritoneal wound repair may be favorably altered by modifying the activities of inflammatory cells to reduce nonspecific tissue injury. Early investigators viewed the acute postinjury phase of healing largely as an "all or none" phenomenon. Their goal was to essentially eliminate the phagocytic component of acute postinjury phase injury by obliterating the inflammatory response to tissue trauma. Powerful immunosuppressive agents (e.g., corticosteroids) were used for this purpose (Replogle, et al, 1966). Other important aspects of peritoneal repair were largely ignored.

Contemporary data suggests that inflammatory and immunocompetent cells have an essential role in the events of reperitonealization extending beyond the acute postinjury phase. Mesothelial and endothelial cells, submesothelial parenchymal cells, macrophages, lymphocytes, and platelets all contribute to the success of wound healing. It has become increasing apparent that the goal of contemporary adhesion prevention regimens should be to redirect the activity of these cellular systems to obtain posttraumatic tissue homeostasis without compromising their essential activity the subsequent phases of fibrinolysis and macrophage-directed reperitonealization. We have described drugs which affect inflammatory/immunocompetent cell function but are not classic antiinflammatory agents to be "immunomodulatory agents". Experiments in animal models for reproductive surgery indicate that perisurgical administration of such diverse agents as calcium channel blockers, pentoxifylline, prostacyclin analogs (iloprost), and bioactive peptides (somatostatin, substance P antagonists) may significantly reduce both primary posttraumatic adhesion formation and reformation.

Calcium channel blocking agents - Preliminary investigations of the effect of calcium channel blockade on peritoneal healing were performed in the hamster uterine horn primary injury model. Sexually mature golden hamsters received a standardized cautery devascularization injury of the left uterine horn at laparotomy. Animals were treated with study medications given by subcutaneous injections. Necropsy was performed two weeks later to assess the extent of primary adhesion formation. Adhesion formation was quantitated using a scoring scale of 0= no adhesions, 4+= most severe. Administration of nifedipine (100-300 μg/kg) (Steinleitner, et al, 1988a), verapamil (100-400 μg/kg) (Steinleitner, et al, 1988b), or diltiazem (100-300 μg/kg) (Steinleitner, et al, 1988c) at 8 hour intervals for three days post-injury resulted in a marked inhibition of primary adhesion formation. The amount of medication administered in these studies corresponded (on a dose of drug per unit body weight ratio) to the standard doses of calcium blockers used in clinical medicine. Similar results were observed in a rabbit uterine horn primary injury model following treatment with verapamil (Steinleitner, 1990a). The these data obtained using calcium blockers from pharmacologically distinct classes suggest that the favorable influence on peritoneal repair is a generalized effect of calcium blockade.

Given that prevention of adhesion reformation is harder to achieve than prevention of primary adhesion formation, we developed a model which more closely mimicked the situation encountered during reproductive surgery (Steinleitner, 1989a). In the rabbit adhesion reformation model, sexually mature New Zealand White rabbits received a standardized adhesiogenic traumatic lesion to the left uterine horn. One week later a laparotomy was performed for evaluation (prescore) and subsequent lysis of adhesions. Following adhesiolysis animals were randomized to treatment with vehicle (n = 10) vs verapamil (2.5

μg/kg/hour, n = 21) delivered via an intraperitoneal Alzet miniosmotic pump. Seven days later rabbits were sacrificed and evaluated in a blinded manner to quantify adhesion reformation (postscore). Mean prescore in control rabbits was 2.9 ± 0.2 and in verapamil treated rabbits was 3.3 ± 0.1, demonstrating that the primary traumatic lesion was effective in inducing adhesion formation. Vehicle treated rabbits had a mean postscore of 3.5 ± 0.3, not significantly different from control. In contrast, verapamil treated rabbits had a mean postscore of 0.5 ± 0.2, consistent with a significant influence on postsurgical peritoneal repair.

Dunn, et al evaluated the potential for synergism between verapamil and intraperitoneally administered tissue plasminogen activator (tPA) for adhesion prevention (Dunn, et al, 1991). These investigators confirmed that perioperative verapamil therapy inhibits postsurgical adhesion formation in the rabbit. Verapamil and tPA were shown to act synergistically to inhibit adhesion formation following a primary traumatic injury.

The mechanisms by which calcium channel blockers act to reduce adhesion formation are presently a matter of speculation. Calcium plays a central role in the regulation of a multitude of cellular and organ level events. Calcium channel blockade has been shown to reduce ischemic cellular injury in a number of animal models (Peck, et al, 1981, Chand, et al, 1984). Calcium channel blockers are potent vasodilators. It is possible that these agents might act to improve perfusion at the tissue level by overcoming reactive vasospasm associated with injury. Release of vasoactive mediators associated with the acute inflammatory response (ie; histamine, prostaglandins E and F) is reduced by calcium channel blockade (Kim, et al, 1985), whereas the release of PGI, a potent vasodilator is stimulated (Mehta, et al, 1986). Verapamil has been demonstrated to limit the increase in vascular permeability accompanying the acute inflammatory response. Inhibition of actinomyosin-mediated "rounding up" of endothelial cells prevents the formation of microscopic pores in small vessels, limiting the exudation of fibrin rich plasma available for clot formation (Mayhan and Joyner, 1984). Penetration of fibrin matrices by fibroblasts, an important mechanism by which gelatinous adhesions become organized, is inhibited in vitro by diltiazem and verapamil (Azzarone, et al, 1985). A similar effect in vivo would be expected to reduce the extent of collagenous adhesion deposition following surgical injury.

Pentoxifylline - Pentoxifylline is a methylxanthine derivative which is presently indicated for the treatment of peripheral vascular disease. Although the initial work with pentoxifylline suggested that it improved microvascular perfusion in diabetics by increasing erythrocyte membrane fluidity, subsequent studies have demonstrated this drug to be a potent immunomodulator. Our initial experiments were performed in the hamster uterine horn primary injury model (Steinleitner, et al, 1989b). Perisurgical treatment with pentoxifylline at doses of 0.1 to 10 mg/kg administered subcutaneously at 12 hour intervals provided significant protection against post-traumatic adhesion formation. A majority of animals demonstrated no gross adhesion formation. In those animals which formed adhesions, bands were generally limited to intrahorn involvement, filmy in nature, and easily separable. Pentoxifylline treated animals at the extremes of the dose response curve (0.001 and 25 mg/kg/12 hours) consistently formed dense adhesions similar to controls. No gross evidence of significant complications such as increased infectious morbidity, bleeding dysfunction or failure of wound healing was noted. A most interesting finding was the observation that delaying the initiation of therapy by as much as 72 hours did not reduce the efficacy of pentoxifylline-mediated adhesion prevention. Initiation of therapy at time points beyond 72 hours resulted in adhesion formation equivalent to control. In the duration of therapy experiment, administration of 3 doses was sufficient to effect a significant reduction in adhesion score. Maximal adhesion prevention was observed with seven or more injections.

Consistent findings were obtained in the rabbit adhesion reformation model (Steinleitner, 1990b). New Zealand White rabbits were randomized to treatment with vehicle (n=12) vs subcutaneous pentoxifylline 2.5 mg/kg/q12h for six doses (n=12) immediately following lysis of established adhesions. Seven days later rabbits were sacrificed and evaluated in a blinded manner to quantify adhesion reformation (postscore). Using a scoring scale of 0= no adhesions, 4+= most severe, the prescore was not different for pentoxifylline and control (3.8 vs 3.9 respectively); however, postscore (0.7 vs 3.7) was markedly reduced by pentoxifylline ($p<0.001$).

Data from the dose- and time-response experiments suggest that pentoxifylline-mediated adhesion prevention is the result of interventions at multiple sites along the adhesion formation cascade. Significant adhesion reduction was observed with administration of three perioperative injections (24 hours of therapy). This finding is consistent with a modulation of acute postinjury inflammatory events. Pentoxifylline is known to influence diverse aspects of leukocyte activation and function including: increased membrane deformability (Schmalzer, 1984), modulation of directed chemotaxis (Sullivan, et al, 1984), reduced oxidative burst and neutrophil degranulation (Bessler, et al, 1986, Slater, et al, 1988), inhibition of cytokine-induced granulocyte adherence to endothelium (Berticchi, et al, et al, 1988), and decreased neutrophil cytotoxicity for endothelial cells (Till, et al, 1988). Pentoxifylline has also been shown to decrease the production of TNF by macrophages (Strieter, et al, 1988) and inhibits the inflammatory action of TNF and IL-1 on granulocytes in vitro (Sullivan, et al, 1988). Data from animal models of infectious (Sullivan, et al, 1984) and noninfectious organ (Bjornson, et al, 1988) insults suggests that pentoxifylline may prevent injury by reducing the inflammatory activities of granulocytes without affecting their bactericidal capability. A similar influence of pentoxifylline upon events occurring in post-surgical tissues might favorably influence mesothelial repair and inhibit adhesion formation.

Results of the initiation of therapy experiment demonstrate that a delay in administration of the drug by as much as 72 hours had no significant effect on adhesion reduction. These data are consistent with an effect of pentoxifylline on later aspects of mesothelial repair. Knox has shown that pentoxifylline enhances in vitro macrophage penetration into clots and production of plasminogen activator (Knox, 1988). Corresponding in vivo activity may result in increased fibrinolysis and release of bound viscera prior to myofibroblast proliferation and reperitonealization.

Iloprost - Given the impact of PGI on platelet-endothelial interactions and fibrinolysis, we theorized that PGI analogs might be useful as a modulator of posttraumatic peritoneal healing. Iloprost, a long lasting PGI analog, shares many properties of the parent compound. Vasodilatory, platelet suppressant, fibrinolytic, and "cytoprotective" activities of iloprost equal or exceed that of PGI (Musil, et al, 1986). Data obtained in the hamster uterine horn primary injury model demonstrate perioperatively administered iloprost to be a potent inhibitor of primary adhesion formation (Steinleitner, in press). This activity occurred in a dose dependent manner with maximal adhesion reduction observed at a dose of 4 mg/kg. The therapeutic index of iloprost in this indication was fairly broad, with significant adhesion prevention occurring over 2 orders of magnitude. Perioperative administration of iloprost did not lead to increased infectious morbidity, failure of wound healing, or obvious bleeding disorders.

While the precise mechanism(s) by which calcium channel blockade, pentoxifylline, and iloprost influence peritoneal healing in these animal models is unknown, these studies clearly suggest that "immunomodulatory" agents have the potential to influence multiple components of the adhesion formation cascade. Such activity would represent a significant improvement over the majority of agents currently being employed or studied for adhesion prevention in which the therapeutic effect is generally limited to intervention at a specific aspect of the inflammation and repair process.

POLOXAMER SOLUTIONS AS BARRIER MATERIALS FOR ADHESION PREVENTION

Although the use of pharmacologic adjuvants has considerable theoretic appeal, application of barrier materials to effect physical separation of injured viscera has emerged as the most effective therapy currently available to surgeons. Characteristics of an ideal barrier material include biocompatibility, absorbability, a neutral or beneficial effect on the events of peritoneal healing, and the ability of the barrier material to serve concomitantly as a local delivery system for pharmacologic anti-adhesion adjuvants.

Poloxamer 407 is a representative of a family of polymers which demonstrate unusual physical characteristics. Aqueous solutions of poloxamer 407 exist as a viscous fluid at 4°C. However, at body temperature poloxamer 407 undergoes a state change to a solid gel. This property is known as "reverse thermal gelation" and is a consequence the micellar configuration of the polymer in aqueous solution.

These properties offered the possibility that poloxamers might be particularly suited to use as barrier materials in infertility surgery. Preliminary experiments by Leach and Henry (1990) demonstrated topical application of poloxamer 407 to be effective in inhibiting primary peritoneal adhesion formation following pelvic trauma in rats. Subsequently, we performed extensive pharmacodynamic studies in the hamster uterine horn primary injury model (Steinleitner, et al, 1991). The anti-adhesion effectiveness of aqueous poloxamer 407 was directly related to the concentration of the material in solution. 30 to 35% (weight/volume) solutions were found to be maximally effective. Animals treated with 35% poloxamer 407 had an average adhesion score of 2.2 ± 0.9 (scale to 6.0) which was equal in effectiveness to treatment with pentoxifylline 2.5 mg/kg. Poloxamer solutions containing less than 30% did not significantly reduce posttraumatic adhesion formation. Increasing the concentration of poloxamer beyond 40% resulted in a material which was difficult to handle and apply to tissues.

The rabbit model was used to evaluate the efficacy of poloxamer 407 for preventing adhesion reformation following adhesiolysis. The experimental method was similar to that employed in our studies with verapamil and pentoxifylline. A primary adhesiogeneic lesion was used to induce adhesion formation in 18 animals. Average prescore for all rabbits at second look laparotomy prior to adhesiolysis was 5.3 ± 0.3 (scale to 6.0). Control rabbits reformed essentially all the adhesions which were resected at the second laparotomy; the average postscore (5.2 ± 0.3) was identical to the prescore in this group. Application of 35% poloxamer 407 following adhesiolysis resulted in a significant reduction in all measured parameters of adhesion formation. Postscore values for adhesion location, thickness, and extent were approximately 50% of the corresponding prescore. Average postscore for poloxamer treated animals was 2.7 ± 0.3. No evidence of infection, failure to thrive, or compromised wound healing was noted in these animals.

The physical characteristics of poloxamer solutions are dependent on ionic strength, pH, and the polarity of other species in solution. Based upon the preclinical data, Mediventures Inc (Grosse Pointe Park, MI) has developed an optimized solution of poloxamer 407 (Flowgel) for use in infertility surgery. Data from the rabbit adhesion reformation model demonstrate this material to be highly effective at inhibiting postsurgical adhesion formation (Steinleitner, in press). Average postscore for poloxamer treated animals was 0. In a blinded comparison of Flowgel with Interceed/TC-7 (Johnson and Johnson, Medical Inc, Arlington, TX) Flowgel was found to be equally efficacious. Preclinical studies of the use of Flowgel in infertility surgery are being initiated at this time.

SUMMARY

Obviously, no single modality will prove to be universally applicable or completely effective at preventing postoperative adhesion formation. Increasing understanding of the pathophysiology of peritoneal healing provides the intellectual basis for the development of specific interventions at critical points along the adhesion formation cascade. We believe that multimodality therapy, including the use of pharmacologic adjuvants such as immunomodulatory drugs and fibrinolytic/anticoagulant agents in conjunction with a barrier material tailored to the specific operative procedure may provide optimal results. Hopefully, developments in the 1990's will provide reproductive surgeons with the means to help patients derive maximal benefit from their reconstructive procedures.

REFERENCES

Azzarone B, Krief P, Soria J, et al: Modulation of fibroblast-induced clot retraction by calcium channel blocking drugs and the monoclonal antibody ALB6 (1985): J Cell Physiol 125:420.

Berticchi F, Proserpio P, Lampugnani MG, Dejana E (1988): The effect of pentoxifylline on polymorphonuclear cell adhesion to cultured endothelial cells, a preliminary report. In: Mandell GL, Novick WJ Jr (Eds): Pentoxifylline and leukocyte function. Proceedings of Pentoxifylline Symposium, Key Biscayne, FL. Somerville:Hoechst-Roussel Pharmaceuticals, pp 68.

Bessler H, Gigal R, Djaldetti M, Zahavi I(1986): Effect of pentoxifylline on the phagocytic activity, cAMP levels, and superoxide anion production by monocytes and polymorphonuclear cells. J Leukocyte Biol 40:747-54.

Bevilacqua MP, Pober JS, Wheeler ME, Cotran RS, Gimbone MA (1985): Interleukin-1 acts on cultured human vascular endothelium to increase the adhesion of polymorphonuclear leukocytes, monocytes and related leukocyte lines. J Clin Invest 2003.

Bjornson AB, Kippenberg RW, Bjornson HS (1988): Effects of pentoxifylline on inflammatory and immunological responses in a guinea pig model of thermal injury. In: Mandell GL, Novick WJ Jr (Eds): Pentoxifylline and leukocyte function. Proceedings of Pentoxifylline Symposium, Key Biscayne, FL. Somerville:Hoechst-Roussel Pharmaceuticals, pp 154-64.

Buckman RF, Buckman PD, Hufnagel H, et al (1976): A physiologic basis for the adhesion free healing of deperitonealized surfaces. J Surg Res 21:76.

Bursch W, Schulte-Hermann R (1987):. Cytoprotective effect of iloprost against liver cell death induced by carbon tetrachloride (CCl_4) or bromobenzene. In: Gryglewski RJ, Stock G (eds):Prostacycline and its stable analog iloprost. Springer-Verlag, Berlin, p 257-68.

Chand N, Diamantis W, Pillar J, et al (1984): Inhibition of allergic and nonallergic histamine secretion from rat peritoneal mast cells by calcium antagonists. Br J Pharmac 83:899.

Craddock PR, Hammerschmidt DE, White JG, et al (1977): Complement (C5a)-induced grannulocyte aggregation in vitro. J Clin Invest 60:260-64.

Dunn RC, Steinleitner AJ, Lambert H (1991): Synergistic effect of intraperitoneally administered calcium channel blockade and recombinate tissue plasminogen activator to prevent adhesion formation in an animal model. Am J Obstet Gynecol, 164:1327-30.

Fukasawa M, Bryant SM, Orita H, et al (1989): Modulation of proline and glucosamine incorporation into tissue repair cells by peritoneal macrophages. J Surg Res 46:166-71.

Harlan JM (1987): Neutrophil-mediated vascular injury. Acta Med Scand 715 (Suppl.):123-9.

Hensen PM, Johnston RB Jr (1987): Tissue injury in inflammation: oxidants, proteases, and cationic proteins. J Clin Invest 79:669.

Hunt TK, Knighton DR, Thakral KK, Goodson WH, Andrews WS (1984): Studies on inflammation and wound healing: angiogenesis and collagen synthesis stimulated by in vivo resident and activated macrophages. Surgery 96:48-54.

Kim YY, Holgate ST, Church MK (1985): Inhibition of histamine release from dispersed human lung and tonsilar mast cells by nicardipine and nifedipine. Br J clin Pharmac 19:631.

Knighton DR, Silver IA, Hunt TK (1981): Regulation of wound-healing angiogenesis - Effect of oxygen gradients and inspired oxygen concentration. Surgery 90:262-70.

Knighton DR, Hunt TK, Scheuenstuhl H, Halliday BJ, Werb Z, Banda MJ(1983): Oxygen tension regulates the expression of angiogenesis factor by macrophages. Science 221:1283-5.

Knox P (1988): Leukocyte-mediated activation of the fibrinolytic pathway and the effects of pentoxifylline. In: Mandell GL, Novick WJ Jr (Eds): Pentoxifylline and leukocyte function. Proceedings of Pentoxifylline Symposium, Key Biscayne, FL. Somerville:Hoechst-Roussel Pharmaceuticals, pp 96.

Leach RE, Henry RL (1990): Reduction of postoperative adhesions in the rat uterine horn model with poloxamer 407. Am J Obstet Gynecol, 162:1317-9.

Liebvoich SJ, Ross R (1976):. A macrophage-dependent factor that stimulates the proliferation of fibroblasts in vitro. Am J Pathol 84:501-13.

Martin BM, Gimbrone MA, Unaure ER, Cotran RS (1981): Stimulation of nonlymphoid mesenchymal cell prolifration by a macrophgae-derived growth factor. J Immunol 1510-5.

Mayhan WG, Joyner WL (1984): The effect of altering the external calcium concentration and a calcium channel blocker verapamil, on microvascular leaky sites and dextran clearance in the hamster cheek pouch. Microvasc Res 28:159.

Mehta J, Mehta P, Ostrowski N (1986): Calcium blocker diltiazem inhibits platelet activation and stimulates vascular prostacyclin synthesis. Am J Med Sci 291:20.

Murray HW, Spitlany GL, Nathan CF (1985). Activation of mouse peritoneal macrophages in vitro and in vivo by interferon-gamma. J Immunology 134:1619.

Musil J, Wilczynska M, Sladek K, Cierniawski CS, Nizankowski R, Szczeklik A (1986): Fibrinolytic activity of prostacyclin and iloprost in patients with peripheral vascular disease. Prostaglandins 1986.

Peck RC, Lefer AM (1981): Protective effect of nifedipine in the hypoxic perfused cat liver. Agents and Actions 11:421.

Polverni PJ, Cotran RS, Gimbrone MA, Unanue ER (1977): Activated macrophages induce vascular proliferation. Nature (Lond.) 269:804-6.

Postlethwaite AE, Lachman LB, Mainardi CL, Kang AH (1983): Interleukin-1 stimulation of collagenase production by cultured fibroblasts. J Exp Med, 157:801-6.

Raftery AT (1973): Regeneration of parietal and visceral peritoneum: an electron microscopical study. J Anat 115:375-92.

Replogle SM, Johnson R, Gross RE (1966): Prevention of postoperative intestinal adhesions with combined promethazine and dexamethazone therapy: experimental and clinical studies. Ann Surg 163:580.

Riches DWH (1988): The multiple roles of macrophages in wound healing. In: Clark RAF, Henson PM, The molecular biology of wound healing. Plenum, New York, 213.

Schmalzer EA, Chien S (1984): Filterability of subpopulations of neutrophils: effect of pentoxifylline. Blood 64:542-6.

Schmid-Schönbein GW, Usami S, Skalak R, Chien S (1980): The interaction of leukocytes and erythrocytes in capillary and postcapillary vessels. Microvasc Res 19:45-70.

Schmid-Schönbein GW (1987): Capillary plugging by granulocytes and the no-reflow phenomenon in th microcirculation. Fed Proc 46:2397-2401.

Schmidt JA, Oliver CN, Lepe-Zuniga JL,, Green I, Gery I (1984): Silica-stimulated monocytes release fibroblast proliferation factors identical to interleukin-1. J Clin Invest 79:1462-72.

Slater K, Wiseman MS, Shale DJ, Fletcher J (1988): The effect of pentoxifylline on neutrophil function in vitro and ex vivo in human volunteers. In: Mandell GL, Novick WJ Jr (Eds): Pentoxifylline and leukocyte function. Proceedings of Pentoxifylline Symposium, Key Biscayne,

FL. Somerville:Hoechst-Roussel Pharmaceuticals, pp 115.

Steinleitner A, Lambert H, Montoro L, Kelly E, Swanson J, Sueldo C (1988) The use of calcium channel blockade for the prevention of postoperative adhesion formation. Fertil Steril 50:818.

Steinleitner A, Lambert H, Montoro L, Kelly E, Sueldo C: Reduction of adhesion formation with perioperative verapamil treatment. Pacific Coast Fertility Society, Palm Springs, CA, 4/88.

Steinleitner A, Lambert H, Montoro L, Swanson J, Sueldo CE (1988) Use of diltiazem for preventing postoperative adhesions. J Reprod Med 33:89.

Steinleitner A, Lambert H, Kazensky C (1989): Calcium channel blockade prevents postsurgical reformation of adnexal adhesions in rabbits. Obstet Gynecol 74:796-8.

Steinleitner A, Lambert H, Kazensky C, Danks P, Roy S (1989): Use of pentoxifylline as an adjuvant to prevent postsurgical adhesion formation: preliminary investigations in a rodent model. J Gynecol Surg, 5:367-73.

Steinleitner A, Lambert H, Kazensky C, Sanchez I, Sueldo C (1990): Reduction of primary postoperative adhesion formation under calcium channel blockade in the rabbit. J Surg Res, 48:42-5.

Steinleitner A, Lambert H, Kazensky C, Danks P, Roy S (1990): Pentoxifylline, a methylxanthine derivative, prevents postsurgical adhesion reformation in rabbits. Obstet Gynecol, 75:926-8.

Steinleitner A, Lambert H, Kazensky C, Cantor B (1991): Use of poloxamer 407 as an intraperitoneal barrier material for the prevention of postsurgical adhesion formation and reformation in rodent models for reproductive surgery. Obstet Gynecol, 77:48-52.

Steinleitner A, Lambert H, Suarez M, Serpa N, Robin B (1992): Reduction of primary post-traumatic adhesion formation with the prostacyclin analog iloprost in an animal model. Am J Obstet Gynecol, in press.

Steinleitner A, Lopez G, Suarez M, Lambert H (1992): An evaluation of Flowgel as an intraperitoneal barrier for prevention of postsurgical adhesion reformation. Fertil Steril, in press.

Strieter RM, Remick DG, Ward PA, et al (1988): Cellular and molecular regulation of tumor necrosis factor-alpha production by pentoxifylline. Biochem Biophys Res Comm 155:1230-6.

Sullivan GW, Patselas TN, Redick JA, Mandell GL (1984): Enhancement of chemotaxis and protection of mice from infection. Trans Assoc Am Physicians 97:337-45.

Sullivan GW, Carper HT, Novick WJ, Mandell GL (1988): Inhibition of the inflammatory action of interleukin-1 and tumor necrosis factor (alpha) on neutrophil function by pentoxifylline. Infect Immun 56:1722-29.

Thiemermann C, Steinhagen-Thiessen E, Schrör K (1984): Inhibition of oxygen-centered free radical formation by the stable prostacyclin mimic iloprost (ZK 36374) in acute myocardial ischemia. J Cardiovasc Pharmacol 6:365-6.

Till GO, Warren JS, Gannon DE, et al (1988): Effects of pentoxifylline on phagocyte responses in vitro and acute and chronic inflammatory responses in vivo. In: Mandell GL, Novick WJ Jr (Eds): Pentoxifylline and leukocyte function. Proceedings of Pentoxifylline Symposium, Key Biscayne, FL. Somerville:Hoechst-Roussel Pharmaceuticals, pp 124-37.

Gynecologic Surgery and Adhesion Prevention, pages 253–259

PREVENTION OF ADHESION FORMATION/REFORMATION WITH THE GORE-TEX SURGICAL MEMBRANE

Charles M. March, M.D., Stephen Boyers, M.D., Robert Franklin, M.D., Arthur F. Haney, M.D., Bradley Hurst, M.D., Eberhard Lotze, M.D. John A. Rock, M.D., Guillermo Rowe, M.D., and William Schalaff, M.D.
University of Southern California School of Medicine, Los Angeles, CA 90033 (CMM)
Duke University Medical Center, Durham, NC 27710 (AFH)
University of Colorado Health Science Center, Denver, CO 80210 (WS)
University of California, Davis School of Medicine, Sacramento, CA 95816(SB)
The Johns Hopkins Hospital, Baltimore, MD 21205 (BH, JAR)
Women's Hospital of Texas and Baylor College of Medicine, Houston, TX 77054 (RF, EL, GR)

INTRODUCTION

The development of adhesions is a leading cause of failure in reconstructive pelvic surgery. Despite the use of corticosteroids, antihistamines, antibiotics, dextran, and oxidized regenerated cellulose (ORC), controlled studies utilizing objective criteria have not identified a universally satisfactory agent. Thus, there is no standard adjuvant therapy for adhesion prophylaxis. Recently, oxidized regenerated cellulose has been studied extensively (INTERCEED (TC7) Adhesion Barrier Study Group, 1989).

GORE-TEX Surgical Membrane (GSM) [W. L. Gore and Associates, Inc., Flagstaff, AZ] is a permanent, inert microporous implant of expanded polytetrafluoroethylene (ePTFE). In 1983, ePTFE was approved for reconstruction of the peritoneum or pericardium. Minimal to no foreign body tissue response has been demonstrated after retrieval of GSM as long as 8.75 years after implantation. Boyers et al. demonstrated the usefulness of ePTFE in reducing primary pelvic adhesion formation in the rabbit experimental model.(Boyers et al, 1988). A preliminary study has demonstrated the efficacy of the Surgical Membrane to prevent adhesion reformation after extensive adhesiolysis or formation after myomectomy (The Surgical Membrane Study Group, 1992).

MATERIALS AND METHODS

After IRB approval twenty-eight subjects entered this study between June, 1989 and July, 1991 at five centers. Subjects were 18 to 40 years old, had a present or future desire for fertility, and signed an informed consent. Group A consisted of eight subjects who had an adhesion score of >11 on either adnexa using the AFS classification of adnexal adhesions4. Prior to adhesiolosis, a site-specific scheme that details type, extent and tenacity was used to grade the adhesions (Table 1). Surgical membranes were implanted over 12 sites.

TABLE 1
SITE-SPECIFIC CLASSIFICATION OF ADHESIONS

	DESCRIPTION	SCORE
EXTENT	NO INVOLVEMENT	0
	<25% SITE INVOLVED	1
	<50% SITE INVOLVED	2
	<75% SITE INVOLVED	3
	<100% SITE INVOLVED	4
TYPE	NONE	0
	FILMY, TRANSPARENT, AVASCULAR	1
	OPAQUE, TRANSLUCENT, AVASCULAR	2
	OPAQUE, CAPILLARIES PRESENT	3
	OPAQUE, LARGER VESSELS PRESENT	4
TENACITY	NONE	0
	ADHESIONS FALL APART	1
	ADHESION LYSED WITH TRACTION	2
	ADHESIONS REQUIRE SHARP DISSECTION	3
TOTAL POSSIBLE		11

Group B consisted of ten patients who had extensive bilateral adnexal adhesions. The left and right sidewall adhesion sites were graded using the site-specific scheme, the adhesions lysed, the resulting defects sized in cm2, and ORC and GMS allocated randomly to the sites.

Group C consisted of ten patients who underwent myomectomy. The GSM were implanted over 18 incision sites. Each center had no more than two designated adhesion assessors who implanted the GSM and who graded all adhesions.

Adhesions were lysed or the myoma(s) removed and the Surgical Membrane was implanted after the size of the defect was assessed. Meticulous hemostasis was achieved before placing any barrier. The GSM was trimmed so that it overlapped the peritoneal defect by at least 1.0 cm (Figure 1). It was secured with at least one non-absorbable suture of 7-0 or 8-0 nylon or polypropylene. In order to insure an unwrinkled implant, further interrupted sutures of 7-0 or 8-0 permanent or absorbable material were placed. ORC was placed over the defect and then moistened so that it would adhere. Prophylactic antibiotics were used for 24 hours. Tubal patency was assessed intra-operatively. The pelvis was then irrigated with sterile, lactated Ringer's solution containing 5000 units of heparin per liter. No other adhesion prophylaxis was used.

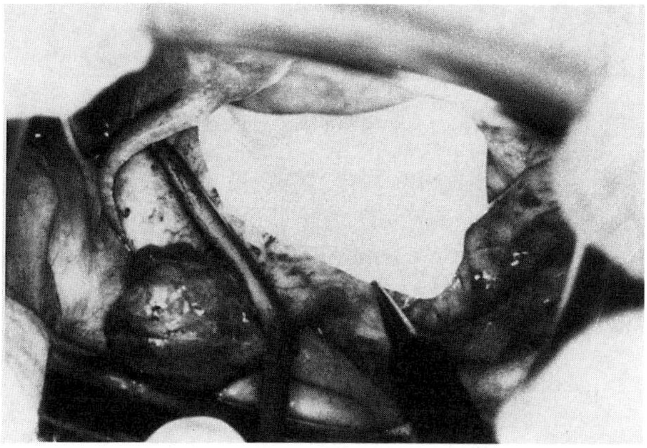

Figure 1. Placement of the Surgical Membrane in the ovarian fossa, just prior to suturing.

One to six weeks later, laparoscopy was undertaken to assess (using the site-specific scheme) and to treat any adhesions and to retrieve the Surgical Membrane.

The adhesion scores were compared using paired non-parametric comparisons. One-way analysis of variants (p=0.065) for all patients indicated that the scores arose from a single population and therefore that the data from all centers could be pooled. A probability of <0.05 was established for statistical significance. RS/1 (Digital Equipment Corp.) was used for statistical analysis.

RESULTS

A total of 28 patients were enrolled in the three study groups. The GORE-TEX Surgical Membranes were implanted in 40 sites for an average of 20.8 + 5.5 days. No complications occurred and laparoscopic removal of the Surgical Membranes was uniformly easy.

Among Group A subjects, the mean score for the site-specific grading scheme for sidewall defects was 10.25 + 0.45 before implantation and 1.42 + 2.19 at the time of laparoscopy (Figure 2).

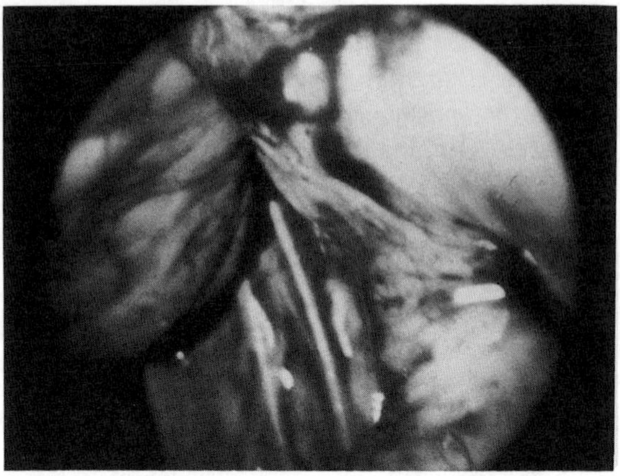

Figure 2. Laparoscopic view of the site shown in Fig. 1, illustrating a lack of adhesions to the site of adhesiolysis.

Thus the site-specific grading scheme demonstrated a significant change (Figure 3). Each site was compared by the total score as well as the component values. All of these two-tailed comparisons were statistically significant, with P<0.0001 (Table 2).

Among those in Group B, the extent of adhesions were similar prior to randomization (10.4 + 0.84 for GSM and 10.7 + 0.67 for ORC) (p<0.99). However, at the time of second-look laparoscopy, the GSM performed significantly better. The adhesion scores for the GSM were 1.70 + 1.89 compared to 4.30 + 3.30 (Table 3, P<0.015).

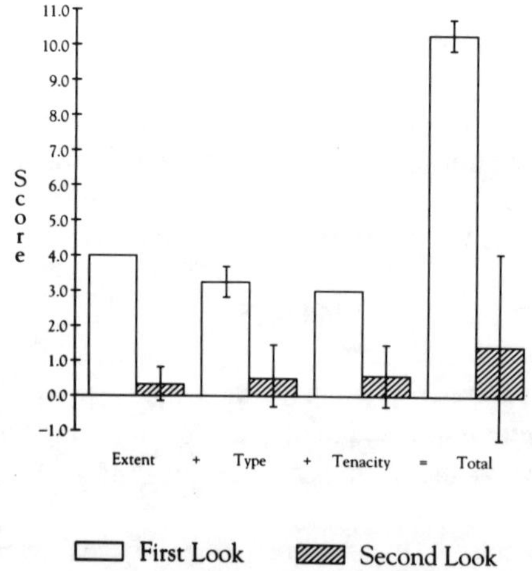

Figure 3. Improvement in site-specific adhesions scores among Group a patients after conservative surgery and placement of the GORE-TEX Surgical Membrane.

TABLE 2
SUMMARY STATISTICS FOR SITE SPECIFIC CLASSIFICATION OF SIDEWALL ADHESIONS AMONG GROUP A SUBJECTS (n=8)

	LAPAROTOMY				LAPAROSCOPY			
	EXTENT	TYPE	TENACITY	TOTAL	EXTENT	TYPE	TENACITY	TOTAL
MEAN	4.00	3.25	3.00	10.25	0.33	0.50	0.58	1.42
STD.DEV.	0.00	0.45	0.00	0.45	0.49	0.90	0.90	2.19
MEDIAN	4.00	3.00	3.00	10.00	0.00	0.00	0.00	0.00

Extent, type, tenacity and total score for adhesion site at Laparotomy versus same at Laparoscopy, 2-tailed Wilcoxon ranked pair Test; $p< .001$ for all pair wise comparisons, n=12 sites.

TABLE 3
COMPARISON OF THE GORE-TEX SURGICAL MEMBRANE (GSM) AND INTERCEED STUDY IN 10 SUBJECTS UNDERGOING ADHESIOLYSIS.

	SITE-SPECIFIC ADHESION SCORES			
	INITIAL LOOK		SECOND LOOK	
	GSM	INTERCEED	GSM	INTERCEED
MEAN	10.40	10.70	1.70	4.30
STD. DEV.	0.84	0.67	1.89	3.30
MEDIAN	11.00	11.00	1.50	5.00

Initial look SM vs Interceed $p< 0.99$
Second look SM vs Interceed $p< 0.015$

TABLE 4
SUMMARY OF STATISTICS FOR SITE SPECIFIC CLASSIFICATION OF ADHESIONS TO 18 MYOMECTOMY SITES IN 10 SUBJECTS

	EXTENT	TYPE	TENACITY	TOTAL
MEAN	0.33	0.33	0.33	1.00
STD. DEV.	0.69	0.69	0.69	2.06
MEDIAN	0.00	0.00	0.00	0.0

Among the 10 patients with leiomyomata (Group C), the mean incision size of the myomas removed was 3.6 cm + 1.5. The mean scores at second look for extent, type and tenacity of adhesions occurring to the myomectomy incision, as well as a mean total score, are shown in Table 4.

Histologic analysis of explanted Membrane showed no tissue ingrowth or adhesion formation (Figure 4). The interstices of the GSM were variably infiltrated with an acellular protein matrix. Occasionally, there were small adhesions to the suture knots that held the GSM in place. There were no infections of the material, while the analysis showed no to a slight foreign body response.

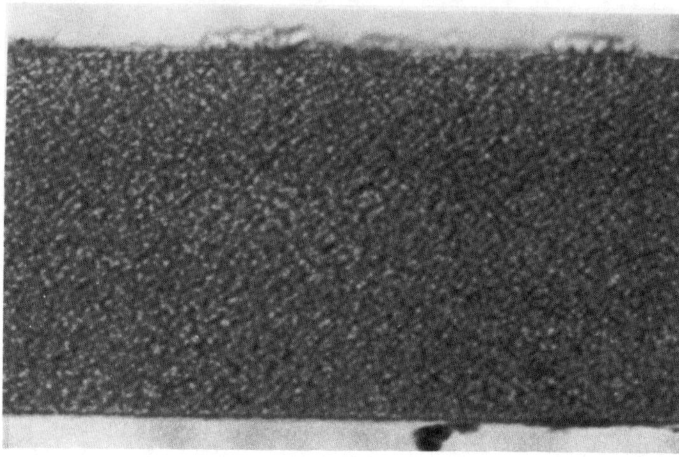

Figure 4. Histological cross-section of Surgical Membrane retrieved from the pelvic sidewall after 22 days. A proteinaceous fluid infiltrates the interstices of the material, but there is no cellular attachment. Originally 100X.

DISCUSSION

Although a variety of agents have been employed to prevent adhesion formation and reformation following conservative infertility surgery, two recurring themes have emerged: the site-specific efficacy of even the most promising agents has never been dramatic and the original favorable results have never been duplicated following widespread clinical use. In this preliminary series of patients, the latter issue was not addressed. However, the reduction in adhesion formation/reformation is dramatic and surpasses that reported previously with other antiadhesion agents.

In addition to the apparent value of the Surgical Membrane, four facts have emerged from this study: experience with a few procedures is necessary in order to gain the facility required to work comfortably; overlap of at least one cm is necessary to prevent adhesion formation to the uncovered edges of raw surfaces; laparoscopic removal can be accomplished with ease; and morbidity did not occur.

All patients enrolled in the study had disease of sufficient magnitude to warrant second-look laparoscopy, and thus removal of the GSM. Because long-term peritoneal placement has not been associated with complications, removal may not be mandatory. If further studies demonstrate efficacy equal to that reported herein, long term implantation may become the acceptable standard.

SUMMARY

Eighteen patients with extensive adhesions and 10 undergoing myomectomy had GORE-TEX Surgical Membranes placed in order to prevent adhesion formation/reformation. At the time of second-look laparoscopy the membranes were removed easily and the extent of adhesion was minimal. Preliminary data from 10 additional patients undergoing adhesiolysis demonstrated that the GSM resulted in significantly fewer adhesions than did oxidized regenerated cellulose. The number of patients in this group will be expanded to insure that this difference is maintained.

REFERENCES

Boyers SP, Diamond MP, DeCherney AH: Reduction of postoperative pelvic adhesions in the rabbit with Gore-Tex$_R$ Surgical Membrane. Fertil Steril 1988; 49:1066-1070.

INTERCEED(TC7) Adhesion Barrier Study Group: Prevention of postsurgical adhesions by INTERCEED(TC7),* an absorbable adhesion barrier: a prospective, randomized, multicenter clinical study. Fertil Steril 1989; 51:933-938.

The American Fertility Society: The American Fertility Society classifications of adnexal adhesions, distal tubal occlusion, tubal occlusion secondary to tubal ligation, tubal pregnancies, Mullerian anomalies and intrauterine adhesions. Fertil Steril 1988; 49:944-955.

The Surgical Membrane Study Group: Prophylaxis of pelvic sidewall adhesions with GORE-TEX Surgical Membrane: A multicenter clinical investigation. Fertil Steril, 1992 (in press)

Gynecologic Surgery and Adhesion Prevention, pages 261-264

CLINICAL EVALUATION OF THE EFFICACY OF HEPARIN-SATURATED INTERCEED FOR PREVENTION OF ADHESION REFORMATION IN THE PELVIC SIDEWALL OF THE HUMAN

Robert L. Reid[1], M.D., Kay Lie[2], M.D., John E. Spence[3], M.D., Togas Tulandi[4], M.D., and Albert Yuzpe[5], M.D.

Departments of Obstetrics and Gynaecology:

1. Queen's University, Kingston, Ontario;
2. University of Toronto, Toronto, Ontario;
3. University of Ottawa, Ottawa, Ontario;
4. McGill University, Montreal, Quebec; and
5. University of Western Ontario, London, Ontario, Canada.

INTRODUCTION

Gynaecologists performing pelvic reconstructive surgery continue to struggle with the problem of post surgical adhesion reformation. In addition to microsurgical techniques, a variety of adjuvants, including medications, lavage solutions, and mechanical barriers have been employed in an effort to minimize recurrence of adhesions. Recently an absorbable barrier, Interceed, composed of oxidized regenerated cellulose has been shown to significantly reduce reformation of pelvic sidewall adhesions in patients undergoing bilateral adhesiolysis[1,2]. Observations from that study indicated that the Interceed barrier did not completely prevent adhesion reformation and, indeed, some adhesions seemed to occur centrally at sites of the Interceed placement. The possibility that blood and fibrin permeating the weave of the material could lead to subsequent collagen deposition and adhesion formation led investigators to consider the potential benefits that might accrue from saturating Interceed with an anticoagulant such as Heparin. Subsequently Diamond et al.[3] were able to show clear evidence of reduction of adhesion reformation in a standardized rabbit uterine horn model in animals receiving Heparin-saturated Interceed in comparison to those receiving Interceed alone.

The present study was undertaken to evaluate the efficacy of Heparin-saturated Interceed for prevention of pelvic sidewall adhesions in the human.

MATERIALS AND METHODS

This multicentre university ethics approved research protocol was conducted on consenting patients 18 years of age or older who were to undergo laparotomy for bilateral lysis of pelvic sidewall adhesions. Adhesions had to involve the posterior/inferior aspect of the broad ligament and cul-de-sac region. Both adnexae had to be preserved at the time of surgery and patients were only included if they agreed to undergo second-look laparoscopy between 10 days and 14 weeks following the initial surgery. Patients were excluded if they were thought to be pregnant, if they had a history or evidence of haematologic or coagulation disorder, if they had received cancer therapy including either drugs or radiation in the past, or if they received any peritoneal instillate or prophylactic medications such as corticosteroids or antiinflammatory agents at the time of surgery. The use of Hyskon at any time during the procedure or for a concurrent hysteroscopy was prohibited as was the use of postoperative hydrotubation.

At the time of initial laparotomy standard microsurgical techniques were employed for adhesiolysis. The area of all raw peritoneal defects was determined by measurement on each side of the pelvis. Meticulous haemostasis was achieved employing needle-point electrocautery, laser, or fine absorbable sutures. Any residual lavage solution was evacuated with suction. At the completion of all surgery an envelope was opened to reveal the randomized treatment assignment. All raw areas on the pelvic sidewall assigned to treatment were to be covered with Heparin-saturated Interceed while the contralateral side remained untreated with either Interceed or Heparin to act as a control. Interceed was either applied dry to the pelvic sidewall and then saturated with a fine spray of Heparin sodium (2 cc of 1000 units per cc) or the barrier was saturated in a dish prior to application. Care was taken to avoid inadvertent contact of the contralateral surfaces with the Heparin-soaked Interceed from the treatment side.

Patients were scheduled for second-look laparoscopy between 10 days and 14 weeks after surgery at which time the type and area of adhesions to each pelvic sidewall was documented. A percentage improvement score was determined by the following calculation: the area of adhesions to the sidewall at laparotomy minus the area of adhesions to the sidewall at laparoscopy over the area of adhesions to the sidewall at laparotomy x 100.

RESULTS

Forty six patients were enrolled in this clinical trial of whom 35 were evaluated at second-look laparoscopy. The primary clinical diagnosis for the 46 patients is shown in Table 1. Seventeen of the 46 patients had had previous pelvic surgery. Eleven patients were not evaluated due to eight dropouts before second look laparoscopy; one required salpingo oophorectomy at the time of the reconstructive procedure; one ectopic pregnancy; and one became pregnant before second look laparoscopy. The treated sidewalls showed an 81% improvement while the sidewalls which received no Heparin-soaked Interceed showed a 60% improvement ($p = .008$). The treatment benefit on the Interceed Heparin-treated side was close to the treatment benefit observed in the previous trial with Interceed alone thus the

Table 1

Primary diagnosis for 46 patients enrolled in trial

Pelvic adhesions	23
Tubal occlusion	7
Pelvic inflammatory disease	13
Endometriosis	2
Other	1

superior result in comparison to the control side could not be specifically attributed to the addition of Heparin. A subsequent study has been conducted to compare Heparin-saturated Interceed barrier to Interceed barrier alone in women with bilateral ovarian adhesions. The results of this study will be reported elsewhere.

The data from the present study do not allow any definitive conclusions about the potential extra benefit of topical application of Heparin using oxidized regenerated cellulose as a delivery vehicle for the prevention of pelvic adhesions. Nevertheless, the results are consistent with previous reports indicating a beneficial effect of Interceed adhesion barrier. Further studies are required to resolve whether Heparin has any synergistic effect in the human.

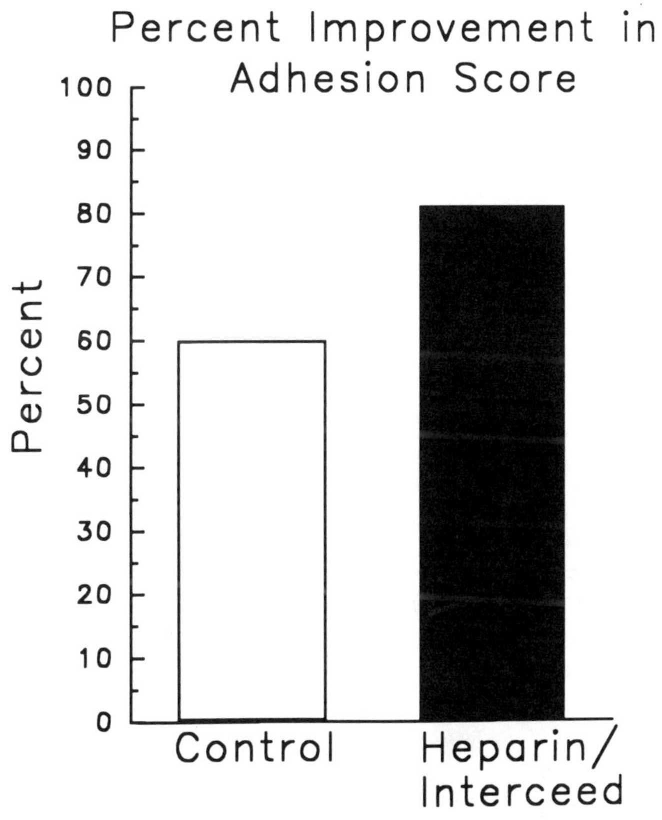

Figure 1.

REFERENCES

1. Interceed (TC7) Adhesion Barrier Study Group: Prevention of postsurgical adhesions by Interceed (TC7) an absorbable adhesion barrier. A prospective randomized multicentreclinical study. Fertil Steril 51:933, 1989.

2. Diamond MP, Linsky CB, Cunningham T, Kamp L, Pines E, DeCherney AH, diZerega GS: Adhesion reformation: reduction by the use of Interceed (TC7) plus Heparin. J Gynecol Surg 7:1, 1991.

3. Use of Interceed (TC7) absorbable adhesion barrier to reduce postoperative adhesion formation in gynecologic infertility surgery. The Japanese Study Group. Obstet Gynecol (Tokyo) 58:1424-1432, 1991.

Index